Younger Skin in 28 Days

Younger Skin in 28 Days

The fast-track diet for beautiful skin and a cellulite-proof body

Karen Fischer

BHSc, Dip. Nut.

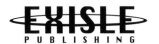

EXISLE PUBLISHING

First published 2013

Exisle Publishing Pty Ltd
'Moonrising', Narone Creek Road, Wollombi, NSW 2325, Australia
P.O. Box 60–490, Titirangi, Auckland 0642, New Zealand
www.exislepublishing.com

National Library of Australia Cataloguing-in-Publication Data:

Fischer, Karen, author.

Younger skin in 28 days : the fast-track diet for beautiful skin and a cellulite-proof body / Karen Fischer BHSc, Dip. Nut.

ISBN 978 1 921966 17 0

Includes bibliographical references and index.

Diet therapy.
Skin—Care and hygiene.
Skin—Aging—Prevention.
Cellulite—Popular works.
Skin—Diseases—Diet therapy—Recipes.
Beauty, Personal.

646.726

Original design concept by saso content & design
Design and typesetting by Tracey Gibbs
Typeset in Minion Pro and Andes Condensed
Printed in Shenzhen, China, by Ink Asia

This book uses paper sourced under ISO 14001 guidelines from well-managed forests and other controlled sources.

10 9 8 7 6 5 4 3 2 1

Disclaimer
While this book is intended as a general information resource and all care has been taken in compiling the contents, this book does not take account of individual circumstances and is not a substitute for medical advice. Always consult a qualified practitioner or therapist. Neither the author nor the publisher and their distributors can be held responsible for any loss, claim or action that may arise from reliance on the information contained in this book.

KAREN FISCHER is a nutritionist and a member of the Australian Traditional-Medicine Society (ATMS). She has a Bachelor of Health Science Degree (BHSc) from the University of New England and a nutrition diploma (Dip. Nut.). In 2008, Karen's bestselling book *The Healthy Skin Diet* won 'Best Health, Nutrition or Specific Diet Book' at the prestigious Australian Food Media Awards. She is also the author of Exisle Publishing's bestselling *The Eczema Diet*. Karen is frequently a guest nutritionist on Australian television and has written health articles for Australian, New Zealand and UK publications. This is her fifth book.

Contents

Introduction

You can be gorgeous at thirty, charming at forty,
and irresistible for the rest of your life.

— Coco Chanel

A wealthy Spanish explorer named Juan Ponce de Leon first heard of the Fountain of Youth when he sailed to South America in 1508.[1,2] Sailors of the 1500s who embarked on long sea voyages were at risk of dying from scurvy so Ponce de Leon brought with him a range of citrus fruits and planted lemon seeds at the ports he frequented — advice which was given to him by the famous explorer Christopher Columbus.

Ponce de Leon settled at San Juan and his slaves built a grand house for him which he named Casa Blanca, meaning 'white castle'. But he was depressed. The years he spent at sea battling harsh weather conditions had wrinkled his skin like an old apple and the decades of drinking liquor had swelled his belly. Then one day, according to legend, he overheard one of his Indian slaves say, 'In Bimini no one grows old.'

'Bimini! What is Bimini?' he asked.

'It is a beautiful island fragrant with flowers that lies far to the north of us. There is a spring of clear water and everyone that bathes in it becomes as young and strong as he was in his best days.'[3]

Ponce de Leon asked around and the fountain seemed to be common knowledge among the slaves. So he made up his mind to conquer Bimini and claim the Fountain of Youth as his own. Ponce de Leon prepared three ships. In 1513, after exploring several islands to no avail, the Spaniards discovered a strange coast where the land was covered with flowers. It happened to be Easter Sunday, or Pascua Florida which meant 'the Feast of Flowers', so Ponce de Leon named the land Florida. The Spaniard planted lemon and orange trees in Florida to protect his men from dying of scurvy. Then he roamed the land, drinking from every clear spring and bathing in many streams and lakes. He did not regain his youth and he eventually gave up the search.

But the anti-ageing fountain played on his mind for many years and so Ponce de Leon returned in 1521 to conquer Florida and establish a Spanish colony. The natives fought back and Ponce de Leon was struck by an arrow. 'Take me back to Spain,' he wailed, 'for I shall never find the fountain of youth.' His ship carried him to Cuba but he soon died from his wound.

Ponce de Leon's search for a miracle natural spring may have been fruitless, but according to historical documents, he did discover a remarkable remedy that could heal the skin and extend life expectancy. It was so revolutionary that it would take the rest of the world more than 200 years to discover this cure and another 100 years before doctors would accept it as a legitimate skin treatment.

Ponce de Leon knew, thanks to his fellow Spanish explorer Columbus who had passed on the remedy, that citrus fruits prevented the skin from falling apart. Suffered by sailors and land-dwellers alike, scurvy was, at the time, a baffling disease where your skin slowly fell apart due to lack of vitamin C in the diet. The first signs were dry skin and mysterious bruising, fatigue and cracked and bleeding lips. As the vitamin C deficiency worsened, the skin would become bumpy and old wounds reopened as the skin's collagen bonds weakened and sufferers eventually bled to death. In fact, in 1595, a Dutch fleet sailed to the East Indies with 249 men, and returned two years later with only 88 survivors because they did not eat enough vitamin C-rich fruits and vegetables.[4]

In 1747, more than 200 years after Ponce de Leon, British surgeon James Lind was credited with discovering the cure for scurvy. It took another 100 years for citrus fruits to be accepted as a legitimate treatment for scurvy around the world and in 1932 vitamin C was isolated as the therapeutic nutrient.[5] And while vitamin C was not the Fountain of Youth originally sought by the Spanish explorer, it was one piece of the anti-ageing puzzle.

Younger skin

The quest for younger skin has been recounted for centuries. The ancient Egyptians had many rituals for beautifying themselves. Cleopatra, the Queen of Egypt, bathed in sour milk which was rich in skin-smoothing lactic acid, and women in ancient Rome rubbed their skin with fermented grape skins (resveratrol-rich remnants from the bottom of wine barrels).[6] Ancient Chinese emperors sent sailors in search of youth-restoring pearls. Today we have botox, lasers and fillers (to name a few) to magically smooth our skin.

I believe everyone has the right to do whatever they like in the quest for beautiful skin so I am not going to admonish the artificial options. We are so lucky to live in an age where many anti-ageing treatments — both natural and artificial — are available if we wish to use them. However, many of us are still searching for that miracle quick-fix — a fountain of youth — that will make us young again, while overlooking one major fact: *your skin is made from the foods you eat.* According to US research, today many Americans still suffer from scurvy (the ancient sailors' disease!) because people are simply not eating enough fruits and vegetables.[7] It's a simple reminder to include healthy food in your beauty regime.

Is avoiding mirrors the answer?

According to UK researchers from the Centre for Appearance Research (CAR), 90 per cent of women don't like the way they look. There are women who also dread looking in the mirror, with 39 per cent saying it brings up negative feelings about themselves. There is even a movement in the United States where women are avoiding mirrors. Mirror fasting — where people cover up all the mirrors in their house and avoid their reflection when out — is not the answer to low self-esteem and it can promote unhealthy self-neglect in some cases.

Your appearance — your weight, your skin, your waistline — gives you valuable clues about how healthy you are on the inside, so it's important to look at yourself for an honest appraisal once in a while. For example, if you have prematurely aged skin it could indicate you are eating too many AGEs — advanced glycation end products — in your diet and some simple changes could create younger skin and potentially increase your lifespan. Sagging skin or poor skin tone can indicate you have a deficiency in the mineral copper. A large waist size can predict diabetes and heart disease risk so being unhappy about your waistline can prompt you to change your diet, which could one day save your life. Loving who you are begins with being honest about what you like and dislike, caring about your feelings (even the bad ones) and then cheering yourself up by taking loving care of yourself.

I wish someone had told me to look after my skin and eat healthy food when I was younger. I spent some of my childhood in Darwin, in a town where it was permanently hot and sunny (except during cyclone season, when it rained). My nose constantly peeled from playing in the sun and my diet was an unhealthy combination of strawberry milkshakes, toast and pies (oh, and I loved hot chips and chocolate mousse). I couldn't comprehend eating a salad. It was no surprise that my first wrinkle appeared by the time I was eighteen. I remember thinking I looked so old!

As I grew up I have wanted one thing above all others — beautiful skin. It is one of the reasons why I became a nutritionist. During and since my teenage years I have suffered from many skin complaints including blemishes on my face and severe dermatitis on my hands, and at one stage, psoriasis covered half my body. I used cortisone cream on my face for many years, which thinned my skin. I was always getting ill and I felt tired all the time so I thought there was something seriously wrong with me. I kept asking my doctor to run tests, which always came back looking okay, and each time he would prescribe *healthy food and exercise* for my ailments. I'm a little bit stubborn and I need scientific proof before I will even consider changing my habits, so I read hundreds of research papers on skin health while I studied nutrition and completed a health science degree. This took more than four years (I told you I'm stubborn) but I'm glad I did.

Since changing my diet I no longer suffer from skin disorders but my quest for younger skin has intensified so researching for and writing this book has been a great joy.

Why 28 days?

Younger Skin in 28 Days is a fast-track program designed for people who have a special occasion coming up such as a wedding, holiday or any date by which you want to look your best. It can be used to complement your current beauty regime, or if you are having a cosmetic procedure you can use this program to supply the nutrients in your diet needed to speed up your recovery and enhance your results.

It is a 28-day program because it takes that long for your body to produce new skin cells in the deeper skin layers and for them to travel to the surface of your skin — so it's literally the beginning of a new you by day 28. It also takes about 21 days to form new habits, so by the end of the program you might automatically continue with some of your healthy new habits.

The program is designed to boost your metabolism and supply all the nutrients needed for skin repair, renewal and maintenance. It can also improve your energy and feelings of wellbeing, and it's healthy for the whole body. There's also plenty of non-diet information to make choosing the right anti-ageing skin care a breeze.

Conditions that can be improved include:

- ✺ premature ageing
- ✺ fine lines and wrinkles
- ✺ dry skin
- ✺ rough or bumpy skin
- ✺ poor skin tone and cellulite
- ✺ mild age spots and hyperpigmentation
- ✺ excessive body odour and bad breath
- ✺ fatigue and sluggishness
- ✺ hypoglycaemia (food related)
- ✺ inability to lose weight
- ✺ abdominal bloating
- ✺ poor immunity to colds and flu
- ✺ candida albicans infestations
- ✺ slow wound healing
- ✺ poor exercise recovery, and much more.

Beauty is not only skin deep — if you look after your skin you will improve your inner health too. More than 200 million people worldwide suffer from osteoporosis, and in women over 45 years of age brittle bones account for more days spent in hospital than many other diseases, including diabetes, heart disease and breast cancer. However, if you look after your skin you won't be one of them. The Younger Skin program can also be used to lower your cholesterol levels and control blood sugar to decrease your risk of type 2 diabetes.

As everyone is unique and you probably have specific desires when it comes to improving your skin, this program can be tailored to suit your needs. For example, if you have stubborn conditions such as cellulite, dry skin or acne you can look up the specific course of action in the table provided at the back of the book. Keep in mind that 28 days is a very short period of time and this program is designed to work fast so be prepared — you will have to do some work every day during the 28 days. But it will be worth it, and you can enjoy younger skin at the end of it.

Beautiful skin enhances people's lives and promotes self-confidence. And I hope at the end you can look in the mirror and feel comfortable in your skin because confidence is one of the most attractive features you can possess. I hope you enjoy the program and I wish you health and happiness on your way to having younger skin.

Karen Fischer

Medical note

If you are taking prescription drugs, undergoing surgery, laser or injections, suffering from an illness, are pregnant or breastfeeding, please consult with your doctor before changing your diet or taking supplements of any kind. The advice in this book does not take the place of advice from your health care professional.

Part 1

Younger skin

Chapter 1

Younger skin

*Wrinkled was not one of the things
I wanted to be when I grew up.*

— unknown

Beautiful skin is a blessing that you take for granted when you are young. It's your largest organ (and the most visible one) and you walk around clothed in it every day of your life. So it helps if you like how your skin looks and feels. Then you grow up, and ageing happens. The skin becomes drier, bumpier and wrinkles appear and you wonder if it's time to let go. You might think: *should I forget about looking good and just accept the inevitable?* However, instead of giving up looking after yourself once you reach a certain age, *now is the time to step up your health and skin care routine, because healthy, younger-looking skin is more than just a pretty façade …*

❀ Your skin acts as a barrier and a filter between the outside world and your insides and it protects your body from invading microbes and fungus.

❀ It helps to regulate your body temperature so you don't overheat and accidentally cook your internal organs.

❀ The skin plays an active role in the immune system, helping to protect you from diseases, bacteria and viruses.

❀ The skin plays a major role in maintaining bone health.

❀ The skin can also show early signs of nutritional deficiencies and indicate that a change in diet is due.

Your skin performs a wide range of important body functions and it plays a vital role in keeping you alive so it pays to look after it. And with today's research and technology it's easier than ever before to keep your skin looking younger for years to come. Let's take a closer look at your skin as it gives us valuable clues on how to look after it.

Upon the skin

The *epidermis* is the outer (or dead) layer of your skin. It is thinnest on your eyelids at .05 mm ($\frac{1}{1000}$in) and thickest on your palms and soles at approximately 1.5 mm ($\frac{3}{50}$in). The epidermis itself contains five layers, which are mostly made up of cells that produce keratin, a tough and fibrous protein that forms a protective layer. The column-shaped cells in the bottom layer push cells into higher layers — *this skin-renewing trip takes about 28 days*. The top layer of the epidermis, the *stratum corneum* (or skin barrier), is made of flat, dead cells that shed about every 2 weeks.

❀ Every 40 minutes you shed about 1 million dead skin cells, and over a lifetime you'll shed enough skin to fill a suitcase.

❀ Between the ages of 30 and 80, the skin's cell turnover rate decreases by 30 to 50 per cent (but you can increase this with the right skin care routine).

Diagram 1: Human skin

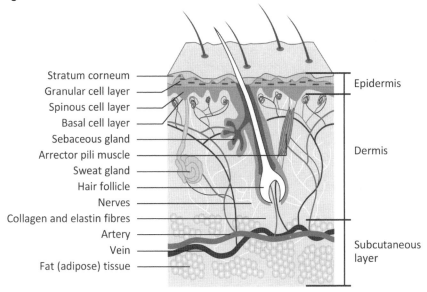

Stratum corneum
Granular cell layer
Spinous cell layer
Basal cell layer
Epidermis
Sebaceous gland
Arrector pili muscle
Sweat gland
Hair follicle
Dermis
Nerves
Collagen and elastin fibres
Artery
Vein
Fat (adipose) tissue
Subcutaneous layer

New skin cells form at the bottom of the epidermis and when they're ready they move towards the stratum corneum. In normal, healthy skin this trip takes about 4 weeks.

When the epidermis is functioning properly, the following youth-preserving properties are at optimal levels:

Properties of healthy skin	Functions	FYI and tips
acid mantle — your skin should have an acidic pH of approx. 5.5	protects the skin from harmful microbes and candida overgrowth	nutrients that promote it: dietary skin lipids, unsaturated fatty acids and amino acids from protein foods;[1] use skin care products that are 'pH balanced'
sebum — made up of oils and fatty acids, secreted from sebaceous (oil) glands	waterproof sealant, moisturises the skin (overactive = acne; underactive = dry skin)	beta-cryptoxanthin, a carotenoid in papaya, red capsicum, paprika and pumpkin (winter squash), increases sebum and skin hydration; zinc and vitamin A normalise overproduction[2]

Properties of healthy skin	Functions	FYI and tips
sweat — produced via sweat glands in the dermis	flushes microbes from the surface of your skin; contains lysozyme, an enzyme that fights bacteria; assists with the removal of waste products from your body	as you age, sweat declines; daily exercise, enough to sweat, gives your skin a natural, healthy glow
skin pigment — formed in the epidermis by melanin and haemoglobin (blood)	helps to protect your skin from UV rays and reduce the risk of skin cancer	as you age, liver spots and uneven pigmentation can occur

The bridge

Interlocking finger-like waves join the epidermis to the dermis, which is the deeper layer of the skin. This important junction allows nutrients and oxygen to travel from the inner layers to the outer layer of the skin so it stays healthy. When hormone levels such as oestrogen decline, the finger-like junctions flatten and nutrient exchange slows, causing loss of elasticity in the skin. However, no matter what your hormones are doing (or not doing) *daily exercise can help to manually improve blood flow to the surface of your skin.*

Deeper skin

The deeper layer of the skin is the *dermis*. It's like the soil in a garden, situated below the surface with the all-important jobs of maintaining the skin's structure and supplying nutrients and fluids. The dermis is a thick layer containing bundles of collagen fibres and coarse elastic fibres made of elastin, which enable the skin to stretch and return to its original shape. The dermis also contains sweat glands, hair follicles, veins and hyaluronic acid which attracts and holds water. Wrinkles appear when changes occur to the deeper layers of the dermis.[3]

When the dermis is functioning properly, the following four youth-preserving properties are at optimal levels.

Collagen

Collagen is like the glue that keeps your skin together. It's an amazing protein structure in the skin that twines in a triple rope-like formation, called a helix, so it is extra strong and durable — on a per weight basis collagen is nearly as strong as steel. More than one-third of collagen is made up of the amino acid glycine, another third is proline and a small proportion consists of lysine and other amino acids. These amino acids are found in protein-containing foods such as fish, eggs, meats, beans, nuts and seeds. For healthy collagen production in the skin, your diet needs to be rich in protein, vitamin C, iron, zinc and manganese. As you age, there is a reduction in collagen fibres, especially in the upper dermis.

Elastin

If you were to pick up an elastic band and stretch it around a jar and then later take it off, the elastic band would snap back into its original shape and size. The elastic fibres within your dermis should also stretch (up to 150 per cent of their relaxed length without breaking) then return to their original shape. Elastin is a protein found within coarse elastic fibres in the dermal layer of the skin, which branch together to give the skin strength and flexibility. Like a lycra swimsuit that loses tautness over time, your skin can lose some of its elasticity during the ageing process.

Hyaluronic acid

In normal skin, glycosaminoglycans (GAGs) such as hyaluronic acid are found between collagen and elastic fibres in the dermal layer. Hyaluronic acid is also found in the epidermis of younger skin but disappears as you age. It is hydrophilic, which means it attracts water, which protects collagen and elastin from becoming rigid.

Smoking cigarettes decreases the amount of hyaluronic acid in your body. You can increase hyaluronic acid naturally by supplying its main building block, glucosamine, in your diet. Magnesium and zinc are also needed to manufacture hyaluronic acid. It's thought that traditional societies who age well do so because their traditional diet, rich in root vegetables, supplies plenty of magnesium and zinc for hyaluronic acid production.

Blood supply rich with nutrients

A healthy blood supply to the skin gives your complexion an attractive, healthy glow. The bloodstream carries oxygen and nutrients to the skin for maintenance, repair and building of new skin cells. As you age, the walls of blood vessels in the dermis become thicker and more rigid, and if your diet (or your digestion) is poor, your skin may not receive enough nutrients. The first indicator is a dull complexion and over time problems such as skin abnormalities, premature ageing and poor wound healing (and skin ulcers in the case of diabetes) can occur.

The cushioning

Beneath the dermis lies the *subcutaneous layer*, which contains fat cells. Your fat cells provide cushioning and insulation to protect the body and plump the skin so it looks younger. As you age, these fat cells get smaller in areas such as the face, and if you are thin your face can age faster because you have fewer fat stores to pad your skin and minimise the appearance of wrinkles.

In areas such as the thighs, bottom and stomach, the opposite can occur. The subcutaneous layer *thickens* (predominantly in women) so fat cells protrude into the dermis and cause the appearance of cellulite.

Cellulite

Cellulite is considered a cosmetic defect, not a disease or a disorder. It appears as lumpy skin and is caused by disordered fat cells in the subcutaneous layer.

Largely thanks to genetics, women have a tougher battle with cellulite. However, female athletes usually have no cellulite, even as they age, and it's from these ladies that we can gain hope and also a bit of insight into how to avoid or reduce cellulite. Research shows that weight loss (if it's required) causes fat cells to retract out of the dermis.

FAQ: 'Why do women get cellulite more often than men?'

Around 5 per cent of men develop cellulite and up to 90 per cent of older women will have it at some point in their life. Women are more likely than men to develop cellulite because they have three main structural differences in the skin:

1. The epidermis or outer layer of the skin is thinner in women (men naturally have tougher skin and women have lovely soft skin).

2. The dermis layer of the skin is a lot thinner in women and this progressively worsens with ageing, eventually allowing fat cells to protrude into this layer.

3. Women have more fat cells and subcutaneous tissue (increased cushioning to help women survive childbirth).

Diagram 2: The skin pinch test

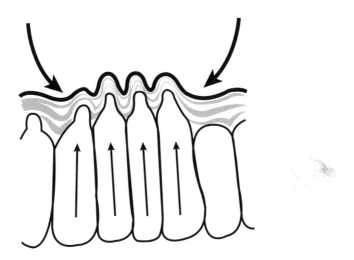

During a pinch test, fat cells can protrude into the dermis in the bottom and thigh region, and occasionally the stomach.

Frequent exercise is one of the keys to minimising or preventing cellulite; another is taking a calcium citrate supplement. Research also shows that massage helps reduce water retention, improve lymphatic drainage and increase collagen synthesis in sufferers of cellulite. Cellulite advice is listed in the Skin Problem Chart on p. 216 and read the calcium information on p. 78.

Skin messengers

Your endocrine system, comprised of your *hormones and glands*, is heavily involved in the ageing process. The endocrine system produces and regulates hormones, which can drastically decline as you age. Hormones are used to regulate growth, mood, metabolism, sexual and reproductive function, and collagen production in the skin, to name a few.

Oestrogens are the main sex hormone in women and they're present in small amounts in men. Oestrogens increase glycosaminoglycans (GAGs) such as hyaluronic acid, which softens and hydrates the skin and helps to maintain structural quality (which is why women have softer skin than men). Oestrogens have anti-inflammatory properties and they play a role in the network of collagen and elastin in your skin, helping to increase collagen production and promote healthy hair.[4]

If you are going through menopause

Menopause is a perfectly normal milestone in a woman's life where menstruation ceases and you are no longer fertile. It begins with peri-menopause where oestrogen levels gradually drop. Low oestrogen levels can promote inflammation and decrease collagen production in the skin, and skin elasticity decreases by 0.55 per cent per year after peri-menopause.[5] Calcium supplementation is essential during menopause as low oestrogen causes calcium deficiency which contributes to loss of skin elasticity. Epidermal ridges also flatten, which increases skin fragility and hampers nutrient distribution in the skin — this can cause your complexion to look dull. However, *this is greatly improved with daily exercise, which flushes the skin with nutrient-rich blood (provided you also eat a healthy, nutrient-rich diet).* For information on treating menopause-related skin problems, refer to the Skin Problem Chart on p. 216.

Chapter 2

The new bad guys in ageing

To understand how to create younger-looking skin, let's look at the main ways you age: these are intrinsic and extrinsic. Your genetics are thought to influence *intrinsic* ageing, such as your hormone levels naturally declining as you age. Skin that ages intrinsically, with little or no extrinsic assaults, is generally fairly smooth with some noticeable expression lines, pigment changes, greying hairs and skin dryness.[1]

Extrinsic ageing, on the other hand, is largely influenced by external factors. These are the habits you can often limit or avoid such as frequent sun exposure, poor diet and cigarette smoking. Extrinsic ageing contributes to deep wrinkles, frown lines, dehydrated skin, rosacea and sallow skin to name a few. Ageing may not be totally avoidable but you can certainly avoid or limit factors that cause extrinsic ageing, including the new bad guys in ageing — molecules called *advanced glycation end products*, also appropriately referred to as AGEs or AGE.

AGEs

AGEs is the new buzzword in ageing research as AGEs appear to be a major factor in skin ageing and have been implicated in diseases such as diabetes and heart disease. Sugars such as glucose are involved as they attach, or cross-link, to proteins in collagen and form the advanced glycation end products. This cross-linking stiffens collagen and elastin fibres and renders them incapable of easy repair.[2] AGEs can also be *consumed in your diet*. They're rich in fried meats and some other foods, and high consumption of dietary AGEs contributes to tissue damage and impaired wound healing of the skin.[3] Another way AGEs can accumulate in the body is via UV radiation from the sun.

Think of AGEs as brownish spots — like sticky toffee — that grab onto collagen when there is lots of sugar in your blood. Not all AGE-rich foods are brown, but when you eat browned foods (from frying and roasting), you're getting a higher dose of AGEs. When your skin goes brown in the sun, AGEs are forming too. Although keep in mind that your skin doesn't necessarily need to go brown to be accumulating AGEs — fair-skinned people are at increased risk due to low pigment and dark-skinned people may have added protection against sun-induced AGEs.

Accumulation of AGEs is associated with:

- ageing
- reduced skin elasticity
- inflammatory skin changes
- yellowing of the skin
- cataracts and other eye problems
- reduced muscle function and strength
- elevated blood sugar levels
- diabetes
- atherosclerosis
- Alzheimer's disease
- Parkinson's disease
- loss of bone density

* loss of muscular mass
* end stage renal disease
* rheumatoid arthritis.[4,5,6,7,8,9]

AGEs accumulate in the dermal layer of your skin partially by attaching themselves to collagen proteins. A collagen fibre normally forms a spring-like coil structure and maintains skin elasticity in combination with elastin fibres. However, when AGEs attach to collagen the cross-links lock the collagen fibres in place and skin elasticity is reduced (See Diagram 3).

Diagram 3: Cross-linking of collagen and AGEs accumulation in the skin

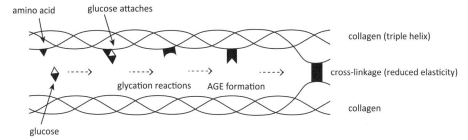

The research ...

* Accumulation of AGEs in the dermis layer of the skin changes the optical characteristics of cells, causing reduced skin transparency and skin yellowing.[10,11]
* AGEs cause damage because of their pro-oxidant and inflammatory actions and the skin can appear red and blotchy.[12]
* AGEs and the cross-linking of collagen cause stiffening of blood vessels and loss of muscle mass and strength as you age.[13]

Glycation — the chemical process that generates AGEs — increases in frequency as you age. There are three main ways AGEs can form *within* your body: the oxidation of glucose caused by free radicals; the peroxidation of fats which are also damaged by free radicals (see 'Free radical skin ageing' on the following page); and via the Maillard reaction.

The formation of AGEs via the Maillard reaction happens in three stages:

1. This is a slow process that relies on sugars being present and the first step takes place within hours of ingesting sugars such as glucose. If the concentration of glucose subsequently declines, this initial reaction is reversible.[14]

2. If glucose stays elevated, the second stage occurs and over a period of days 'early glycation products' form. This phase is reversible if your blood sugar levels decline (if you give your body a break from consuming sugars and processed carbohydrates which supply high glucose).

3. If the early glycation products accumulate, over a period of weeks they form cross-link proteins *which are not reversible*. The brownish end-products are called AGEs, and they literally age you (refer to Diagram 3 on the previous page).[15]

Free radical skin ageing

A slice of cut apple soon begins to brown; raw meat past its use-by date turns brown and rust appears in an old car due to a process called *oxidation*. In fact, corrosion, rust and oxidation all mean the same thing. Oxidation in the human body can be caused by AGEs and by molecules called free radicals. Free radicals are best described as unstable molecules or 'one-armed thieves' — they have an 'arm' (an electron) missing and they are looking to fill this missing space by stealing an electron from a nearby cell in your body. This causes oxidation of the cell, resulting in DNA damage or cell death.

Your body produces free radicals all the time, when you move and eat, and they are a normal part of the making and functioning of your cells so they are partly unavoidable. However, *excess* free radicals can become a problem and lead to rapid ageing of the skin.

Excess free radicals can be caused by:

❋ smoking
❋ poor diet

- glycation and ingesting foods rich in AGEs
- inflammation
- microbes (such as bacteria) entering the skin
- direct exposure to UV sunlight.

Free radicals set off a chain of events in the body that degrades collagen and elastic fibres. They also trigger the overproduction of melanin, leading to mottled skin pigmentation and other common signs of ageing.[16]

Super heroes in the skin

While free radicals can't be totally abolished, free radical damage in the skin can be greatly reduced by a diet and skin care regime rich in *antioxidants*. Antioxidants include vitamins A, C and E, alpha-lipoic acid, anthocyanins, beta-carotene, lycopene, zinc, selenium, coenzyme Q10 and resveratrol to name a few.

Antioxidants protect your skin cells by donating one of their electrons to a free radical — so the free radical can no longer damage a nearby skin cell. By stopping the chain reaction of destruction caused by free radicals, antioxidants become oxidised themselves (it's better them than you!).

Antioxidants are supplied by a healthy diet rich in vegetables and exotic grains and fruit, and antioxidant-rich skin care products also have a protective effect on the skin.[17]

The research ...

- The antioxidant carnosine protects against glycation as it blocks the cross-linking of sugars with collagen.[18,19]
- Lab studies showed that alpha-lipoic acid reversed collagen glycation due to its antioxidant action and blood sugar level-reducing effect.[20]
- A study found that cinnamon, ginger, cloves, marjoram, rosemary and tarragon all have a protective effect against AGEs because they contain protective phenolic antioxidants.[21]
- Antioxidant flavonoids such as luteolin, quercetin and rutin, from onions and other vegetables, inhibit various stages of AGE formation.[22]

AGE Questionnaire

Fill out the following questionnaire to see if you're exposed to increased levels of AGEs. Circle the most correct answer (YES / SOMETIMES / NO) for each question. Your score for each answer is in brackets. For example in question 2, if you eat puffed/flaked breakfast cereal three times a week your answer is YES and your score is 10. Write your score in the space provided to the right.

YES = weekly or daily
SOMETIMES = monthly or occasionally
NO = never or very rarely

Part A

1. **How old are you?**

   under 20   (0)

   20 to 34   (10)

   35 to 44   (30)

   45 to 54   (40)

   55 to 64   (50)

   65 or above   (60)   _____

2. **Do you eat commercial breakfast cereal? (These are the cereals that are crunchy, crispy, toasted or puffed, not including raw oats or porridge.)**

   YES (10) SOMETIMES (5) NO (0)   _____

3. **Do you eat toasted bread *with* butter or margarine?**

   YES (15) SOMETIMES (10) NO (0)   _____

4. **Do you eat toasted bread with *no* butter or margarine?**

   YES (5) SOMETIMES (2) NO (0)   _____

5. **Do you like to overcook your toast so it is burnt on the edges?**

   YES (10) SOMETIMES (5) NO (0)   _____

6. **Do you eat fish and/or other seafood?**

   YES (10) SOMETIMES (5) NO (0)   _____

7. **Do you eat chicken that is fried, baked, stir-fried, roasted or grilled? (If you *only* eat chicken that is *poached* or *boiled* give yourself 10 points)**

   YES (15) SOMETIMES (10) NO (0)   _____

8. **Do you eat red meat, such as beef, steak, mince, chops and lamb?**

   YES (18) SOMETIMES (12) NO (0)   _____

9. **Do you eat pork, such as pork chops, bacon, ham, roast pork with crackling?**

   YES (18) SOMETIMES (12) NO (0)   _____

10. **Do you eat fried foods such as fish and chips, chicken nuggets, fish fingers, spring rolls, hot chips, etc?**

    YES (24) SOMETIMES (15) NO (0)   _____

11. **Do you roast, grill, fry or barbecue animal protein foods such as red meat, eggs, seafood and poultry using butter, margarine or vegetable oil of any kind (such as canola, olive, sunflower, coconut, etc)?**

    YES (20) SOMETIMES (12) NO (0)   _____

12. **Do you consume dairy products including milk, cheese, yoghurt, butter, iceblocks (ice lollies) and ice-cream?**

    YES (15) SOMETIMES (10) NO (0)   _____

13. **Do you eat pastries, toasted muesli bars, doughnuts or other toasted or browned bakery items?**

    YES (15) SOMETIMES (10) NO (0)   _____

14. **Do you eat bacon, sausages or hot dogs?**

    YES (22) SOMETIMES (15) NO (0)   _____

15. **Do you eat deli meats such as ham, devon, turkey, salami or Spam?**

    YES (22) SOMETIMES (15) NO (0)   _____

16. **Do you eat pizza or fast-food hamburgers?**

    YES (24) SOMETIMES (15) NO (0)   _____

17. **Do you add sweetener, including artificial sweetener, sugar, honey and other sweeteners, to foods or beverages such as coffee or tea, cereals or desserts? (NO is worth 5 points to account for natural fruit sugars and glucose from some vegetables.)**

    YES (20) SOMETIMES (10) NO (5)   _____

18. **Do you overeat or are you considered overweight?**

    YES (20) SOMETIMES (10) NO (0)   _____

19. **Do you have diabetes or any of the following: high blood sugar, Alzheimer's disease, cardiovascular disease, Parkinson's disease, end stage renal disease, rheumatoid arthritis, cataracts or other degenerative eye diseases?**

    YES (28) NO (0)   _____

20. **Do you drink more than three glasses of alcohol per week?**

    YES (20) SOMETIMES (15) NO (0)   _____

21. **Do you smoke cigarettes?**

    YES (22) SOMETIMES (18) NO (0)   _____

22. **Do you tan your skin through sun exposure or sun beds, or do you spend prolonged time in the sun without sunscreen? (NO is worth 10 points to allow for incidental sun exposure.)**

    YES (30) SOMETIMES (20) NO (10)   _____

    Add up your total score part A: _____

Now fill out part B ...

Part B

1. **How often do you exercise?**

   Daily   (10)

   3–6 days/wk   (5)

   1–2 days/wk   (2)

   Rarely or never (0)   _____

2. **How often do you eat purple fruits and vegetables? These include eggplant (aubergine), blueberries, red cabbage, red onion, purple carrots, purple mixed lettuce, etc.**

   Daily   (10)

   3–6 days/wk   (5)

   1–2 days/wk   (2)

   Rarely or never (0)   _____

3. **How often do you eat salads or steamed vegetables? (a serving size of at least 1 cup)**

   Daily   (10)

   3–6 days/wk   (5)

   1-2 days/wk   (2)

   Rarely or never (0)   _____

4. **How often do you eat raw oats or porridge with fruit?**

   Daily   (5)

   3–6 days/wk   (3)

   1–2 days/wk   (1)

   Rarely or never (0)   _____

5. **How often do you use fresh lemon and lime in drinks, cooking, meat marinades, etc?**

   Daily   (10)

   3–6 days/wk   (5)

   1–2 days/wk   (3)

   Rarely or never (0)   _____

6. **How often do you drink antioxidant-rich teas such as ginger, chai (leaf tea, not powdered chai latte), green tea, peppermint or other herbal teas?**

    Daily (5)

    3–6 days/wk (3)

    1–2 days/wk (1)

    Rarely or never (0) _____

7. **How often do you add cinnamon, cloves or curry powder to your meals?**

    Daily (10)

    3–6 days/wk (5)

    1–2 days/wk (3)

    Rarely or never (0) _____

8. **Do you have naturally dark skin that is resistant to wrinkles and sun damage?**

    No (0)

    Olive skin, Italian, etc. (10)

    Darker skin, African American, African, Indian, etc. (20)

    Add up your total score part B: _____

Now minus your Part B score from your Part A score. For example, if your Part A score was 120 and your Part B score was 75 then your final score would be 45. Your aim on this program is to get your final score as close to 0 as possible. This book will show you how to achieve this. This 0 point indicates low AGEs but keep in mind that AGEs also accumulate as you age, so the older you are the more careful you have to be with your diet and lifestyle.

A quick recap

- Advanced glycation end products (AGEs) are obtained in three ways: they are formed inside the body (due to the natural ageing process and/or the presence of sugars), they accumulate from sun exposure, and they are supplied by your diet.
- Low AGE diets reduce inflammation and oxidative damage.
- Meats, cheeses, fast food and fats contain the highest dietary AGEs.
- Vegetables, fruits, beans and wholegrains are low in dietary AGEs.
- High cooking temperatures and longer cooking times increase AGEs in foods.
- Cooking with liquids and at lower temperatures greatly reduces the formation of AGEs.
- Processed or takeaway/takeout foods contain more AGEs than raw or homemade foods.

Chapter 3

The Dirty Dozen

When it comes to sabotaging your skin, there are a range of factors that can fast-track wrinkling, mottled pigmentation and other signs of ageing. The Dirty Dozen — aptly named as AGEs are brownish in colour — includes activities that elevate AGE formation and foods that promote glycation, the chemical process that creates AGEs. The Dirty Dozen also includes foods that are rich sources of dietary AGEs, which attack collagen and contribute to organ, blood vessel and tissue damage.

The build-up in the body of too many AGEs is linked to diabetes, heart disease and problems with kidney function, and studies also suggest AGEs can harm the immune system and promote arthritis. You may not be able to prevent the biological ageing process (which involves some AGE formation and hormonal changes, and so on) but research shows you can simply eat fewer AGEs to improve your health, skin and longevity.[1] Here are the top factors, the Dirty Dozen, that increase AGEs in the body.

1. Sugar

While some health experts say sugar is an empty calorie food that is harmless in moderation, it appears they may be mistaken. If you want younger-looking skin, new research suggests you skip the sugar and choose healthier options. Sugar consumption contributes to loss of skin elasticity and can trigger the appearance of acne and premature wrinkles. A diet high in sugar may also shorten your lifespan. Scientists from the University of California in San Francisco reported excess sugar consumption is indirectly responsible for 35 million deaths annually worldwide because it significantly increases the risk of AGE-related diseases including diabetes and heart disease.[2]

The research ...

❋ Sugars such as glucose attach to collagen and elastic fibres and form advanced glycation end products. This cross-linking stiffens collagen and elastin fibres, making them difficult to repair.[3]

❋ A low-sugar diet reduces the sugar level within the skin.[4]

There are a range of antioxidant nutrients, such as vitamin C and resveratrol, which can break down some types of AGEs in the body. However, the bad news is there is no agent that can break down the most common AGE, *glucosepane*, which is made when glucose attaches to collagen. Glucosepane levels are ten to 1000 times higher in human tissue than any other cross-linking AGE and *the only way to decrease levels of this harmful molecule is to reduce sugars in the diet*.[5]

On average, Americans consume 27.5 teaspoons of hidden (and not so hidden) sugars every day, according to the US Sugar Association. The annual sugar consumption in most Western countries is a staggering 50 kilograms per person (that's 50 large bags of sugar).[6] Australians, on average, consume 42 kilograms of sugar annually — a daily intake of 28.8 teaspoons (or 115.4g) of sugar, which is far too high and incredibly ageing on the skin.

The following is a list of sugars commonly found in processed food products and recipes:

- agave nectar
- barley malt
- beet sugar
- blackstrap molasses
- cane sugar
- caramel
- corn syrup
- corn sweetener
- corn syrup solids (in baby formulas)
- crystalline fructose
- dextrin
- dextran
- dextrose
- d-mannose
- ethyl maltol
- Florida Crystals
- fructose
- fruit juice
- galactose
- glucose
- golden syrup
- HFCS
- high-fructose corn syrup
- honey
- lactose (milk sugar)
- malt syrup
- maltodextrin
- maltose
- mannitol
- maple syrup
- molasses
- panocha
- rice malt syrup
- sorbitol
- sucrose
- treacle.

FAQ: 'What about artificial sweeteners; are they a healthy alternative to sugar?'

Artificial sweeteners include aspartame, saccharine, sucralose and acesulfame potassium and Americans consume more than 10 kilograms (24lb) of artificial sweeteners per person each year. However, researchers have found that artificial sweeteners can lead to *increased* hunger and weight gain as they stimulate the release of the hormone insulin, which causes the accumulation of body fat.[7] There are also concerns about the long-term safety of consuming large amounts of these artificial chemicals. *Artificial sweeteners are not a healthy alternative to sugars and they are not a part of the 28-day program.*

FAQ: 'Are fruit sugars bad for me?'

Fruit contains fruit sugars such as fructose, which can be used by the body to form AGEs. However, avoiding fruit is not the answer to long-term health — quite the opposite. Most fruits are rich in important antioxidants, which protect against AGEs and free radical damage and lower your risk of diseases. A diet devoid of fruit *causes the antioxidant levels in your skin to plummet* and this puts you at increased risk of diseases such as skin cancer and scurvy, plus it can leave you more vulnerable to sunburn and premature ageing. It's important to consume two to three pieces of fruit daily for good health.

FAQ: 'Carbohydrates are broken down into glucose, so should I avoid all carbs in order to avoid sugars?'

Some glucose in the diet is essential for mental function and energy, so total carbohydrate avoidance is not recommended and it can be harmful to your health in the long term. But there are some carbs your body could do without. Unhealthy carbohydrate foods that are overly processed and supply your body with too much glucose and *too quickly* are the ones to avoid — such as white flour, white bread, biscuits, cakes and other high GI foods. These spike your blood sugar and increase AGE formation.

Others are essential to good health. Lower GI carbohydrates — sweet potato, peas, rolled oats and some other wholegrains — give your body a *steady and gradual* supply of glucose, which is the 'food' your brain uses for mental function and it's your body's main source of energy. Without this slow and steady supply you could have energy crashes and sugar cravings, and you would feel foggy brained and incredibly tired (and relying on coffee and stimulants to function). Wholegrain carbohydrates including rolled oats, spelt and quinoa also give your body an important supply of fibre for bowel health — without enough dietary fibre you would be frequently constipated and more likely to suffer skin breakouts. Some, such as red quinoa and sweet potato, are also a rich source of antioxidants to fight AGE formation.

For younger skin, avoid the unhealthy and overly processed carbohydrate foods and opt for the low GI and wholegrain varieties; stop adding sugar and other sweeteners to your foods; and if you crave something sweet opt for fresh fruit.

2. Not wearing a hat

Research shows that frequent UV exposure is the number one cause of wrinkles but you don't need a study to confirm this — just look at the skin on your bottom (or an area that has not seen the sun) and compare it to your hands and you will see a remarkable difference in skin quality. Wrinkles are mostly found on sun-exposed skin — the face, chest, arms, knees and hands.

Today's children attending primary school in Australia have a 'No hat, no play' rule so they will probably grow up with younger skin than previous generations. However, it's never too late to start protecting your skin from the sun. By the time you're eighteen, your skin has only been exposed to less than 25 per cent of your lifetime UV dose, which means that *most* of your UV-induced skin damage transpires during adulthood.[8]

The research ...

❀ Sun exposure causes the formation of AGEs in the skin, which paralyse collagen fibres and reduce skin elasticity.[9]

❀ In normal skin, glycosaminoglycans (GAGs) are found between collagen and elastic fibres to offer support and hydration. After chronic sun exposure, GAGs move away from these fibres and hang in a different location so the skin becomes drier and prone to wrinkling.[10]

✳ Sun exposure to the skin triggers the appearance of matrix metalloproteinases (MMPs), which degrade collagen and elastic fibres and play a role in skin ageing.[11] The good news is that a mixture of antioxidants, beta-carotene and lycopene in the diet, consumed on a daily basis, can decrease harmful MMPs (but they can't fix all signs of sun damage).[12]

The majority of sun damage occurs not while you're at the beach or on a boating trip (when you are most likely slathered in sunscreen and wearing a hat), it happens during incidental activities. When waiting for your child at the school gate, while driving your car, mowing the lawn, walking to the local shop, getting the mail — these activities and more, account for *two-thirds of your sunlight exposure*. There is no better solution than to become a hat person and wear a hat daily in order to protect your face.

This may feel weird at first but you will soon find your comfort zone if you have a variety of hats to suit different occasions. Remember, it takes 21 days for new habits to stop feeling weird and start feeling natural.

For younger skin, you will need at least three hats: one fashionable wide-brimmed hat or something to suit special occasions; one sports cap for exercise; and another hat to suit your daily outfits and activities. Hats, especially wide-brimmed ones, protect your face and, over the long term, they will shave *years* off your skin's appearance. For men, try on a felt fedora, a classic hat favoured by celebrities such as Johnny Depp, or buy a straw fedora for the summer months. For casual outings or for outdoor work, nothing protects like a wide-brimmed straw hat or Australian-made Akubra, but a baseball cap will suffice.

Tip: go for quality and something that you love because a hat can't save your face if it's sitting in the cupboard.

3. Barbecued steak (and other red meats)

If you want to eat a food that lengthens your lifespan and fights wrinkles then don't throw a steak on the barbecue. According to a 'Food Habits in Later Life' study of 2000 people over the age of 70, the participants who frequently ate red meat had more skin wrinkling than those who rarely consumed it.[13] Animal-derived foods that are high in protein and fats, especially red meat and deli meats, are rich in wrinkle-promoting AGEs and cooking causes new AGEs to form. In contrast, low protein and low fat foods such as vegetables, fruits and wholegrains contain relatively few AGEs even after cooking.[14]

The research ...

- Red meat contains high levels of AGEs before cooking and these skin-sabotaging molecules increase during cooking.[15]
- Of all the foods tested, steak cooked with olive oil contains the most AGEs, closely followed by plain cooked steak. Of the red meats, lamb contained slightly fewer AGEs.[16]
- High intake of red meat is associated with higher levels of toxic nitrosamines or N-nitroso compounds — and the amounts are comparable to those supplied in cigarette smoke.[17,18] White meat, such as chicken and turkey, does not cause higher levels of N-nitroso compounds in humans.[19]

However, wrinkles can be the least of your problems if you frequently eat meat. A study of more than 120,000 people revealed that eating red meat — any amount and type — significantly increases the risk of premature death from cancer and heart disease.[20] Researchers from the Harvard School of Public Health concluded that eating as little as 85 grams (3oz) per day of unprocessed red meat increases the risk of death by 13 per cent. Frequent consumption of processed meats such as bacon and hot dog sausages increases the risk of premature death by 20 per cent — the same as if you smoked cigarettes.[21]

The same study found that eating a handful of nuts instead of eating pork or a beef meal reduces the risk of dying by 19 per cent. You are 14 per cent safer if you substitute a red meat meal for one containing chicken or wholegrains. If you swap lamb for legumes once a week you are 10 per cent better off, and choosing a fish dish instead of red meat reduces the risk of dying by 7 per cent.[22]

AGE content in protein foods

Carboxymethyl-lysine (CLM) and methylglyoxal (MG) are two of the many types of AGEs that are associated with markers of disease and are elevated in patients with diabetes and kidney disease. The following table lists a range of common protein foods and shows the content of AGEs of the CLM variety only.

Content of dietary AGEs in foods[23]

Protein foods	Dietary AGEs in kilounits (kU) per 100g (3½oz)
canned tuna, in water	452
tofu, raw	788
skinless chicken breast, poached/cooked in casserole or soup with added lemon or tomato (acidic ingredient)	682
skinless chicken, parcel-baked with lemon	1047
pork chop, pan-fried (7 mins)	4752
roast beef	6071
steak, grilled/broiled	7478
steak, barbecued or pan-fried in olive oil	10,058

For younger skin, reduce the amount of AGEs consumed as much as possible. As a guide:

- ❊ foods considered low-AGE contain 0–99 kU per 100g
- ❊ low–medium AGE foods contain 100–999 kU per 100g
- ❊ high AGE foods contain 1000–4999 kU per 100g
- ❊ very high AGE foods contain 5000+ kU per 100g.

You can realistically *halve* your daily intake of AGEs if you avoid red meat, prepare your chicken, tofu or seafood (protein) meals by cooking with moist heat — such as by making soups, casseroles and stews — and by ensuring you eat plenty of vegetables. Instead of frying, roasting or grilling/broiling — all of which use high heat and greatly increase AGE production — try lemon poaching, parcel baking or marinating protein foods such as chicken and fish as these methods of cooking produce less than one-quarter of the dietary AGEs of frying.[24]

4. Cheese (and other dairy products)

Consuming dairy products increases your risk of wrinkles and sun damage according to a study of 2000 elderly Australians.[25] The article, published in the *Journal of the American College of Nutrition*, revealed that people who were most wrinkled were the ones who frequently consumed butter, ice-cream or full fat milk. A week of eating ice-cream every night is enough to see visible changes in the skin. And it's no wonder as ice-cream is packed with sugar, saturated fats, milk sugars and additives.

The research ...

- ❊ The pasteurising and homogenising of dairy products, especially butter and cheeses, causes the formation of AGEs, which may partially explain why frequent dairy consumption is linked to wrinkle formation.
- ❊ Dairy consumption increases the risk of acne and researchers suspect this could be due to the animal hormones and bioactive molecules found in milk products.[26]
- ❊ High calcium intake from dairy products blocks the absorption of iron and zinc, which are essential minerals for collagen-production in the skin.
- ❊ Cheeses, especially parmesan, are rich in dietary AGEs and fat-rich spreads such as butter, margarine and mayonnaise are some of the richest sources of dietary AGEs.[27]

Cheese	Dietary AGEs in kilounits (kU) per 100g (3½oz)
cottage cheese, 1% fat	1453
mozzarella, reduced fat	1677
Swiss cheese	4470
brie	5597
feta	8423
American cheese, white	8677
parmesan, grated	16,900

For younger skin, avoid dairy products for at least 28 days. After 28 days, continue to avoid AGE-rich butter, margarines and cheeses. Dairy alternatives are listed on p. 72.

5. Cigarettes

Smoking cigarettes can dramatically alter your physical appearance — the photos on Australian cigarette packs are testament to that. Smokers with a history of heavy smoking are five times more likely to have wrinkles than non-smokers.[28] However, as the advertisements say, every cigarette is doing you harm. Just one cigarette causes the constriction of blood vessels, which hampers blood flow to your skin.[29] This leads to the dull complexion, wrinkled and dehydrated skin and sores that won't heal that are common with long-term smoking.

The research ...

- ❋ Smoking decreases vitamin C levels in the body and it affects the body's ability to form healthy collagen in the skin.[30,31]
- ❋ Tobacco contains high concentrations of wrinkle-promoting AGEs.[32]
- ❋ Cigarette smoke induces metalloproteinases (MMPs) in the skin and MMPs play a role in skin ageing.[33,34]

❋ Smoking causes numerous dermatologic conditions including poor wound healing, premature skin ageing, squamous cell cancers, psoriasis and hair loss.[35]

❋ A staggering 93.7 per cent of sufferers of hidradenitis suppurativa — chronic skin inflammation with blackheads, red bumps and lesions that can enlarge and weep — are smokers or were previous smokers.[36]

For younger skin, enrol in a quit program today.

6. Not exercising

Too busy to exercise? It could be costing you your looks and weakening the health of your whole body. Wounds heal slower in older adults who don't exercise and the risk of skin infection is high when wound healing is delayed.[37] Exercise helps your body remove toxins and waste and it flushes the skin with lysozyme-rich sweat, which kills microbes that can cause skin inflammation. Exercise also flushes the skin with nutrient-rich blood, giving your skin the building materials it needs for cell maintenance and renewal. But what is most exciting about exercise and health is the effect it has on glycation and AGE formation.

The research ...

❋ Frequent exercise reduces advanced glycation end-product formation so it has a protective effect against dietary AGEs and sugar-induced AGE formation.[38]

❋ Exercise significantly speeds up wound healing in older adults.[39]

❋ Frequent moderate exercise reduces inflammation, normalises glucose metabolism and improves renal function in patients with diabetes.[40]

As you age, hormone levels decline and your skin receives fewer nutrients and less oxygen as a result of hampered blood supply. This can leave the skin looking sallow, and inflammation, rashes and other signs of ageing are accelerated. *For younger skin*, do some form of exercise every day to boost nutrient circulation to the skin. Exercise lessens the appearance of cellulite, and daily moderate- to high-impact exercise can prevent cellulite over the long term. Soft sand jogging or walking can work wonders. Speak to a personal trainer if you are unsure of what the best forms of exercise are for your body type, level of health and age.

7. Alcohol

Have you ever woken up after a night of drinking and found your face marked with an imprint from your bed sheets? Alcohol consumption severely dehydrates your skin and causes wrinkle formation, which can take hours to normalise. As you age, alcohol-induced wrinkles can occur on your face and chest, giving them an aged appearance.

Frequent alcohol consumption causes nutritional deficiencies — especially zinc, which is essential for collagen formation — and if left untreated deficiencies can lead to a range of skin diseases, infections and premature wrinkles.

The research ...

* People who frequently drink alcohol have elevated AGEs in the body.[41]
* Alcohol consumption accelerates oxidative stress in the body (causing structural weaknesses, increased cell death and tissue damage), which enhances the formation of AGEs and stiffening of collagen in the skin.[42]
* People who frequently drink alcohol can have multiple nutritional deficiencies, such as vitamin C and zinc deficiencies, which reduce skin elasticity and cause sagging skin.[43]
* The elevation of AGEs in people who frequently drink alcohol might be caused, in part, by the deficiency of vitamins.[44]

According to Australia's Cancer Institute in New South Wales, we may have overestimated the health benefits of alcohol consumption. The heart-protective effects from consuming small amounts of alcohol only relate to people over the age of 45 years, and the health benefits of consuming alcohol only outweigh its damaging effects in mature women over the age of 65.[45]

For younger skin, abstain from drinking alcohol for 28 days and limit alcohol consumption in future.

8. Takeaway and fast food

Takeaway or takeout meals are a special treat for many Western families (some indulge more than others) but is your Friday fish 'n' chips night ruining your skin? Fast-food outlets use oils that are heated repeatedly and these oils change form when cooked at high temperatures. They become harmful trans fats, which behave like saturated fats in the body, and it's estimated that trans fats cause one out of every five heart attacks in the United States, according to the Harvard School of Public Health. Trans fats cause inflammation and increase the risk of heart disease, obesity, strokes, diabetes and high cholesterol. Fried foods that are cooked with quality heat-resistant oils are less prone to trans fats but they pose a different problem: they are rich in AGEs which attack skin collagen, decreasing skin elasticity. The following table details the amount of AGEs in various fast foods and anything over 1000kU per 100g is considered high or very high.

Takeaway and fast foods	Dietary AGEs in kilounits (kU) per 100g (3½oz) (unless specified)
soy burger	55
French fries	1522
2 eggs fried in margarine	2749
potato chips	2883
tofu, fried/sautéed	4723
toasted cheese melt, open-faced	5679
chicken nuggets (90g/3oz)	8627
2 slices pizza (180g/6½oz	12,285
hamburger (standard size 216g/7½oz)	16,850

While poaching, steaming and boiling foods are methods that use lower heat, up to 100°C (212°F), other cooking methods use temperatures that greatly increase AGE formation in foods:

* ❋ grilling/broiling   225°C (437°F)
* ❋ deep-frying   180°C (356°F)
* ❋ roasting   177°C (350°F)
* ❋ oven-frying   230°C (446°F)

The searing heat used in cooking methods such as baking and oven-frying cause browning and this increases AGEs formation in foods, especially ones that are rich in protein and fats. Fried foods from fast-foods outlets — especially the oven-fried foods such as chicken nuggets and pizza — are incredibly rich in AGEs and they are literally ageing you.

For younger skin, you know what to do: avoid fast foods and use gentler cooking methods such as poaching, boiling, stewing, soup-making and steaming — and don't forget raw foods as they are the lowest in AGEs.

9. Burnt toast

A piece of toast or a bowl of cereal might be standard breakfast food, but is breaking the fast with crispy processed foods damaging your skin? Buttered slices of toast contain AGEs that increase in frequency the more burnt the toast is, so you might want to turn down the setting on your toaster and opt for healthier spreads. And it's not just toast that is a problem: processed breakfast cereals containing toasted flakes, crispy biscuits or puffed grains contain their share of AGEs too.

The research ...

* ❋ Commercial breakfast cereals, toast and biscuits which have been baked *until crispy* contain ten times the amount of dietary AGEs as untoasted bread (without butter or margarine).[46]
* ❋ Wholegrain breads contain up to 70 per cent fewer AGEs than processed white bread.[47]

❇ Wholegrains don't generally increase AGEs in the body unless they have been toasted or cooked to a crisp or buttered.[48]

❇ Untoasted breakfast cereals, such as rolled oats or porridge, reduce the risk of heart disease and premature death, but intake of refined breakfast cereals does not have the same protective effect.[49]

Carbohydrate foods	Dietary AGEs in kilounits (kU) per 100g (3½oz)
white rice, boiled	9
oatmeal, cooked (porridge)	14
bran flakes	33
wholemeal bread (untoasted, no butter or margarine)	53
wholemeal bread, toasted	137
white Greek bread, toasted	607
corn chips (average of 2 brands)	886
croissant	1113
pretzel sticks	1600
doughnut, chocolate iced	1803
Rice Krispies breakfast cereal	2000
toasted cereal bar	2143
2 slices white toast (60g/2oz), butter (10g/⅓oz)	2712
waffle, toasted	2870
cookie, biscotti	3220

Compared with protein foods such as red meat, butter and fast foods, carbohydrates contain fewer dietary AGEs. However, carbohydrate foods cause an AGE problem another way: they supply glucose and cause it to spike in the blood, which can set off a glycation reaction that can lead to irreversible AGE formation.

For younger skin, opt for low GI wholegrain foods such as oats, untoasted muesli, porridge, red or black quinoa (not white as it's high GI), basmati rice, wholemeal pasta (such as spelt pasta) or choose wholegrain spelt bread and keep the toaster setting on low.

10. Deli meats

Deli meats, including ham, salami, devon, sausages and bacon, may be flavour rich but they're also rich sources of advanced glycation end products. Deli meats largely owe their moreish flavours to saturated fats, artificial flavour enhancers and smoking methods that cause the AGE content to skyrocket. And there is plenty of research to suggest that deli meats are not only harmful to your skin but may also shorten your lifespan.

The research ...

❁ Researchers from the Harvard School of Public Health found that frequent consumption of processed meats such as bacon and hot dog sausages increases the risk of premature death by 20 per cent — the same as if you smoked cigarettes.[50]

❁ Processed meats contain very high levels of AGEs and toxic nitrosamines, which increase the risk of cancer, heart disease and diabetes.[51]

Deli meats	Dietary AGEs in kilounits (kU) per 100g/3½oz (unless specified)
smoked salmon	572
deli ham, smoked	2349
smoked turkey breast, seared	6013
bacon, microwaved 3 mins	9022
2 pork sausages, 180g (6½oz), microwaved 1 min	10,698
2 strips of bacon, pan-fried (50g/2oz)	11,000
2 beef sausages (frankfurters), 180g (6½oz) boiled 5 mins	13,472
2 beef sausages (frankfurters), 180g (6½oz) grilled/broiled 5 mins	20,286

For younger skin, swap AGE-rich deli meats for fresh foods cooked on low heat.

11. Butter and margarine

The types of fats you eat can show on your face — consume too many saturated fats, from foods such as butter and red meat, and you can either develop pimples or get dry, prematurely aged skin (depending on your genetics, you could end up with both). Margarines are problematic too as they contain varying levels of polyunsaturated and monounsaturated oils that have been tampered with in order to make them solid and spreadable. Some brands contain trans fat, which behaves like saturated fat in the body. Margarines also contain preservatives and other artificial additives and they are rich sources of omega-6 which are over-consumed in the West. Research shows families who frequently use margarine are more likely to have children who develop eczema by the age of two.[52,53] Both butter and margarine are rich sources of dietary AGEs and both can age your skin.

The research ...

- ❉ Butter and margarine top the AGE-rich list, closely followed by processed or 'light' olive oil.
- ❉ Olive oil that is *first cold-pressed* is far lower in AGEs because it has not been heated during the manufacturing process.[54]
- ❉ Avocado, which is unprocessed and rich in monounsaturated fat, is far lower in AGEs than other fat-rich spreads.[55]

Fats, spreads	Dietary AGEs in kilounits (kU) per 10g (⅓oz)
avocado	157
mayonnaise	940
extra virgin olive oil, first cold pressed	1004
olive oil, processed with heat	1200
margarine	1752
butter	2648

12. Overeating

Research shows that overweight people have elevated AGEs in their blood.[56] One in four Australian adults is obese according to the Australian Bureau of Statistics, and 37 per cent are overweight. Overeating (and under-exercising) can not only greatly increase the amount of AGEs you accumulate in your body, it can shorten your lifespan and lead to all sorts of health problems including heart disease and diabetes. The modern Western diet is partly to blame, as diets rich in sugar and artificial sweetener can trigger overeating, and excess consumption of red meat and fried foods is favoured.

The research ...

- High protein diets greatly increase the burden of AGEs in the body and can cause kidney damage.[57]
- Elevated blood levels of AGEs in obese and overweight adults can be successfully reduced by a low calorie diet.[58]
- If you reduce your dietary intake of AGEs by 50 per cent you can reduce levels of oxidative stress and lessen deterioration of insulin sensitivity and kidney function as you age.[59]

A low-calorie diet is recommended for weight loss if you are obese or overweight but it is not necessary if you are within the healthy weight range for your height. If you are unsure if you are within a healthy weight range, ask your doctor.

A quick recap

❋ Reduce the amount of sugars consumed in your diet.

❋ Your face is your fortune — protect it with a hat.

❋ Abstain from drinking alcohol for 28 days.

❋ Don't burn your toast.

❋ You can significantly reduce your intake of dietary AGEs by reducing intake of solid fats (butter and margarine), beef and other fatty meats, dairy products and fried foods, and by increasing your consumption of fish, legumes, vegetables, fruits and wholegrains.[60]

❋ You can potentially halve the amount of AGEs by changing the way you prepare food, and using medium- to low-heat cooking methods.

❋ Instead of frying, roasting or grilling, use low-AGE cooking methods such as poaching, boiling and steaming and make soups, curries, stews and casseroles.

Swap this	for that
red meat	*skinless* chicken (marinated with lemon)
pork/bacon/ham	marinated fish or tofu
deli meats	raw nuts and seeds
sausages	seafood or beans
beef mince	turkey mince cooked with liquids or tomato
cow's milk	non-dairy milks, e.g. organic soy milk
butter/margarine	hummus dip or avocado
cheese	raw nuts and seeds
processed breakfast cereal	rolled oats or porridge (oat or quinoa)

A note on teas and coffee

You may have noticed there was no mention of coffee in this chapter. Coffee contains beans which have been roasted so coffee is a source of AGEs, however (and thankfully) not enough to put coffee in the Dirty Dozen. But coffee does contain caffeine so I recommend you *limit coffee intake to one or two cups per day* (and avoid coffee that has been brewing in a pot for hours as this is rich in AGEs). Or opt for black tea and herbal teas as they are practically AGE-free.

Keep in mind that most teas, especially black tea, contain tannins which bind to iron and can cause iron deficiency if you frequently drink teas with your meals or close to meal times. So if you choose to drink tea have it in between meals and ensure you are consuming enough iron for good health (see iron information on p. 87).

Coffee, black tea, green tea and chai tea contain caffeine and are therefore a source of acid in the body, but you can enjoy two cups a day to boost your antioxidant levels in the skin. Naturally caffeine-free herbal teas such as ginger, peppermint and lemon are excellent choices.

Chapter 4

Top 12 foods for younger skin

The best weapon against skin ageing is your fork — eating the right foods supplies your skin with the nutrients it needs to produce new collagen, fight AGEs and look healthier and younger. This chapter gives you the top 12 anti-AGE foods for younger skin.

1. Purple salad leaves

You might know that eating dark leafy greens is good for your health but a plate of purple foods — or red or even black — could be the best prescription for your skin. Chances are if you have ever bought a mixed salad you have eaten a range of purple salad leaves. The purple, black or red pigments in vegetables are caused by a group of antioxidants called anthocyanins, which makes purple foods (and red and some black foods) more nutritious than light green salad leaves. Purple salad leaves include purple osaka, radicchio (red chicory, Chioggia), red coral lettuce, red mignonette, red oak leaf and red leaf lettuce (which is purple at the tips).

Other types of purple or red leafy plants include red cabbage, purple basil, purple pak choi, purple kale and baby beet greens. Recipes include Mixed Salad Wrap (p. 197), Sweet Potato Salad (p. 200), and Mango and Black Sesame Salad (p. 205).

What are anthocyanins?

Anthocyanins are powerful antioxidant flavonoids. They're also *nature's sunscreen* — a protective pigment giving fruits, vegetables (and some grains) their purple, blue, red or black hues. Think eggplant, cherries, blueberries, pomegranates and black rice (purple corn and purple carrots too). There are more than 300 types of anthocyanins found in nature. Prehistoric and traditional diets were abundant in berries and other anthocyanin-rich foods but today's modern Western diets are relatively low in them.

A German study found that diabetics who took a supplement of 600mg of anthocyanins daily for 2 months had a reduction in abnormal collagen production.[1]

Anthocyanins:
- are powerful antioxidants, therefore protecting blood vessels from oxidative damage
- can reduce high blood sugar levels in people with diabetes
- help neutralise the enzymes that can destroy connective tissue in the skin
- can repair damaged proteins in blood vessel walls, and their anti-inflammatory properties activate the production of type II collagen
- have the ability to block metalloproteases (MMP-1, MMP-9), which degrade collagen and elastic fibres and play a role in skin ageing
- offer mild UV protection[2]
- have anti-cancer properties and purple pigmented foods such as eggplant (aubergine) may be beneficial for those undergoing cancer treatment and chemotherapy
- have anti-inflammatory properties and help to protect against glycation and AGE formation.

2. Red quinoa

Quinoa (pronounced keen-wah) is a healthy gluten-free seed and, although a seed, the ancient Incas referred to it as *the mother of all grains*. It's similar to a true grain as it's rich in carbohydrates but it's also abundant in antioxidants, folate, iron, magnesium, zinc, dietary fibre and protein. Both *red quinoa* and the black variety are lower in carbohydrates than white quinoa and owe their rich colour to anthocyanins. As with many carbohydrate-rich foods, quinoa can affect your blood sugar levels (white quinoa has a high glycaemic index but the darker varieties have a lower GI) so favour red quinoa and have it with cinnamon, which will help keep your blood sugar levels steady.

You can use quinoa as an alternative to rice: just boil it with vegetable stock for 20 minutes, or try the delicious Quinoa and Pomegranate Salad (p. 203), Oregano Chicken Sticks (p. 208) or Quinoa Porridge (p. 171; see also 'How to cook quinoa' on p. 209).

What is the glycaemic index?

The glycaemic index, or GI, is a measure of how foods affect your blood glucose levels. You might know these as 'blood sugar levels'. Protein and fats don't usually affect blood sugar; it is specifically a food's *carbohydrate content* that causes a spike in the sugars present in your blood (which is why you can feel a pleasant energy high when you eat sugar or high GI foods such as potato chips).

Low GI foods fall in the range of 0–55, medium GI is 56–69, and high GI foods are above 70. For example, white bread has a GI of at least 70, Australian sweet potato is rated 44 (but kumera from New Zealand is 78), and basmati rice is 58, which is a better choice than jasmine rice which has a GI of 109. Low GI foods, such as most vegetables, are digested at a slower rate so they release glucose into your bloodstream gradually. This is ideal, and will help you to feel fuller for longer and give you a steady supply of energy in between meals. High GI foods such as puffed cereals (including puffed rice and amaranth), white bread (especially Turkish flat bread) and other white flour products are digested rapidly and flood your bloodstream with large amounts of glucose.

In the short term, the high GI foods give you a 'high' feeling as glucose boosts energy, but like all highs it does not last and you'll soon crave that glucose buzz and feel hungrier than normal, so overeating can result. High GI foods can also lead to energy slumps where you crave sugar as a quick fix. Over time, these glucose highs can damage blood vessels, stress the pancreas (the organ that dishes out insulin), cause weight gain, prematurely age the skin and cause an increase of AGEs in the body. So when eating carbs, favour lower GI choices such as basmati rice or sushi rice (instead of high GI jasmine or brown rice); sourdough bread (instead of regular white bread); and add cinnamon to meals such as oats, quinoa and curry dishes as cinnamon has a blood sugar-lowering effect (more on this later).

3. Black sesame seeds

Black sesame seeds are similar to the white variety, except the black ones are unhulled and far more nutritious. The black variety are superior to white sesame seeds because they naturally taste as if they're toasted so you don't have to fry them to get that delicious nutty flavour. They are rich in protective anthocyanins, which give the seeds their blackened hue, and are a source of protein, magnesium and zinc, which are essential for healthy skin and new collagen formation. Sprinkle some black sesame seeds onto salads or rice dishes. See Sushi Rolls with Black Sesame (p. 186), Mango and Black Sesame Salad (p. 205), Beetroot and Carrot Salad (p. 181), Guava and Rocket Salad (p. 188), and Sweet Potato Salad (p. 200).

4. Blueberries

Berries contain anthocyanins, which give blueberries their dark purple pigment. The other antioxidants present in this superfood include resveratrol, vitamin C and vitamin E, which work together to give blueberries their strong anti-glycation properties.[3,4,5] Research shows the unique range of phenolic compounds in berries significantly reduces generation of harmful AGEs.[6,7] And there is promising lab research showing how resveratrol has the ability to inhibit chemical-induced skin cancers, so this particular antioxidant is of great interest to researchers in anti-ageing and skin care fields.[8]

Best of all, fresh blueberries are delicious and they make a great addition to Omega Muesli (p. 169), Berry Porridge (p. 170) and desserts, or add frozen blueberries to Moisture Boost Smoothie (p. 164). It's easy to grow your own blueberries — first check to see if the climate is suitable in your area. The home-grown varieties are even more delicious than the store-bought varieties.

5. Pomegranate

Pomegranate is an exotic red fruit and an important source of antioxidants, including anthocyanins and vitamin C. The bioflavonoid antioxidants present in pomegranate seeds help to protect against free radical production and inflammation, which can damage cells.[9] Commercially prepared pomegranate juice (which has a little of the rind tannins present) has an antioxidant activity three times greater than that of green tea or red wine (and fresh-squeezed pomegranate juice has twice the antioxidant activity).[10]

Ellagic acid is an important flavonoid antioxidant found in pomegranates, blackberries, cranberries, pecans, raspberries, strawberries, grapes and walnuts.[11] Studies show that ellagic acid prevents AGE formation and, according to researchers, this anti-glycating effect could help control AGE-mediated diabetic symptoms and AGE-related eyesight problems.[12] Pomegranate also contains gallic acid, which inhibits the accumulation of advanced glycation end products and protects collagen.[13]

Pomegranate seeds are best eaten by adding them to salads such as Quinoa and Pomegranate Salad (p. 203) or drink half a cup of commercial pomegranate juice (pure, no added sugar). For tips on how to de-seed a pomegranate see 'How to choose and de-seed a pomegranate' on p. 204.

6. Red onion

Most onions, including red onion, are rich in quercetin, a potent antioxidant which protects against oxidative damage and AGE formation.[14,15,16] However, red onion has the added benefit of containing coloured anthocyanins which lower blood sugar and activate the production of collagen in the skin. Red onions have strong antifungal, anti-inflammatory and antibacterial properties thanks to allicin, an organic sulfur compound which gives onions their unique taste and smell.

Korean researchers tested 25 common plants and red onion was found to have the most potent array of antioxidants and anti-glycation activity, which protects against AGE formation in the skin.[17] Red onions have anti-diabetic properties and consuming 100g (3½oz) of raw red onion reduces blood glucose levels to within a healthy range. However, simply add any amount of raw or cooked red onion to soups, casseroles and salads to make an anti-AGE meal. Recipes include the Anti-ageing Broth (p. 176), Shiitake Vegetable Soup (p. 178), Spiced Sweet Potato Soup (p. 175) and Moroccan Lemon Chicken (p. 198).

7. Red guava

Guava is one of the most nutritious fruits with up to 300mg of vitamin C per 100g (3½oz) — six times more vitamin C than oranges — and it is a rich source of lycopene, which helps to protect the skin from sun damage and skin cancer. Guavas contain ellagic acid and anthocyanins, which offer strong antioxidant protection and inhibit the formation of advanced glycation end products.[18] The fruit has the added benefit of lowering blood sugar.[19]

Rich in gallic acid and quercetin, guava leaf extract (a herbal extract) strongly inhibits high blood sugar and the formation of AGEs.[20] The active compounds in guava also help to restore anti-ageing antioxidant enzymes including superoxide dismutase (SOD) and glutathione peroxidase, making guava a super anti-ageing fruit.[21] Recipes include Papaya Cups with Lime and Guava (p. 159) and Guava and Rocket Salad (p. 188), or have them as a snack — the skin is edible, just wash them and remove the seeds. If guava is not in season buy cherries.

8. Yellow curry powder (turmeric, cumin, ginger)

Yellow curry powder contains a range of powerful spices that protect your skin from AGE-related damage. *Turmeric* gives curry its yellow–orange colour thanks to the presence of curcumin. Curcumin has been widely researched because it has an exciting spectrum of therapeutic activities including anti-inflammatory, antioxidant, anti-cancer, antibacterial, antifungal, antiviral and blood-thinning properties.[22] In lab studies, curcumin improves collagen formation and accelerates wound healing; it inhibits AGE formation and prevents collagen cross-linking and damage.[23,24]

Cumin seeds, often used in the form of ground cumin, add a delicious mild flavour to curries. Cumin has been touted as an 'anti-diabetic spice' and it's almost as potent as cinnamon when it comes to lowering blood sugar levels. Cumin is also capable of reducing oxidative stress and inhibiting AGE formation and cross-linking of proteins making it a wonderful addition to any anti-ageing diet.[25]

Ginger — often used as fresh ginger root or ground ginger — is another common curry spice that inhibits glycation, and has an anti-inflammatory effect on the skin.[26] Ginger also boosts levels of important anti-ageing enzymes glutathione (GSH) and superoxide dismutase (SOD), which play a role in longevity and younger skin. Recipes include Eggplant and Cauliflower Curry (p. 189), Winter Spiced Dahl (p. 190), Curry Naan Bread (p. 193), Moroccan Lemon Chicken (p. 198) and Steamed Chicken and Mint Meatballs (p. 210).

9. Cloves

Of all the herbs and spices, cloves are the best at preventing AGE formation according to lab studies.[27] Cloves are unopened flower buds and have been highly prized since ancient times. In 207 BC cloves were used to sweeten the breath of Chinese emperors.[28] Cloves' medicinal properties include antifungal, antiviral, anti-inflammatory, antimicrobial, anti-diabetic and anti-thrombotic activity. According to research, a drop of clove oil has antioxidants 400 times more powerful than blueberries. Eugenol, the key ingredient in cloves, reduces inflammation by blocking series 2 prostaglandin formation.[29]

Clove tea is beneficial for eliminating intestinal worms, candida albicans and other parasites — but be warned, a high dose of clove can cause a temporary bowel flushing effect which helps with the elimination process. Cloves are best used in curries in the form of *garam masala*, a popular spice mix made from ground cloves, cinnamon, cumin, black pepper and cardamom. And cloves are often in chai tea — favour the leaf or tea bag varieties (not powdered chai, which is rich in sugar and powdered dairy milk). Clove recipes include Chai Tea with Clove (p. 167), Watercress Soup (p. 182), Eggplant and Cauliflower Curry (p. 189) and Moroccan Lemon Chicken (p. 198).

10. Cinnamon

Cinnamon is the second best spice (after cloves) at inhibiting AGE formation. And it has the added benefit of containing protective phytochemicals such as cinnamaldehyde, which reduces blood sugar levels, promotes satiety (so you're less likely to overeat) and lowers LDL cholesterol, which is the bad kind.[30] What is most exciting and useful about cinnamon is its potent ability to slow the absorption of carbohydrates in the bowel, so your body needs less insulin to control blood sugar, making cinnamon a super anti-ageing spice. This is good news as it means you can confidently enjoy quality wholegrain carbs in moderation if you add a dash of cinnamon to the meal.

Buying cinnamon: what to look for

All types of cinnamon are fine to use in moderation but *Ceylon cinnamon* is the top choice. Chinese cinnamon and cassia cinnamon — the most common varieties used in ground or powdered cinnamon — are rich in coumarin which can be toxic in very high doses but fine to consume in small amounts such as those recommended in cooking. If you like to use a lot of cinnamon, look for Ceylon cinnamon, which is usually only available as whole cinnamon sticks known as quills. When ground at home, Ceylon cinnamon is sweeter tasting and more aromatic than the other varieties. Spotting authentic Ceylon cinnamon is easy — the bark is softer and thinner than other types of cinnamon and Ceylon cinnamon quills also roll up in one direction, whereas other types of cinnamon bark roll from both directions and meet in the centre like a scroll. Ceylon cinnamon is easy to break apart so you can grind it in a seed or coffee grinder or use a mortar and pestle to make it into lovely fragrant ground cinnamon.

However, any form of cinnamon is better than none so buy what you can. Add it to breakfast cereals, porridge, smoothies and quinoa recipes, or use the spice mix garam masala in curries as it contains both cinnamon and cloves. Recipes include Omega Muesli (p. 169), Quinoa Porridge (p. 171), Moisture Boost Smoothie (p. 164), Spelt Flat Bread (p. 192), Eggplant and Cauliflower Curry (p. 189), Oregano Chicken Sticks (p. 208) and Shiitake Vegetable Casserole (p. 202).

11. Lemons and limes

Lemons and limes are two of the best fruits for younger skin. Lemons and limes are not only highly alkalising, they also supply vitamin C and when they are added to meals they significantly reduce AGE formation.[31] Lemons and limes are acidic before digestion but once in the body they become highly alkalising and great for the skin.

If you like eating protein foods such as chicken or fish, coat it in a marinade that includes lemon or lime juice to reduce AGEs formation during cooking.[32] Recipes include Tamari, Lycopene and Lemon Marinade (p. 151), Ginger and

Lime Dipping Sauce (p. 157), Flaxseed Lemon Drink (p. 165), Parcel Baked Fish (p. 184), and Steamed Fish with Lime and Ginger (p. 212).

Acid-alkaline balance

So what does it mean when foods are 'acid-forming' or 'highly alkalising'? This refers to how a food affects your pH. Your food does more than stop the hunger pangs and boost your energy; once your meal is digested it releases either an acid or an alkaline base into your bloodstream. To be healthy, your blood needs to be slightly alkaline, at a pH between 7.35 and 7.45, and your body will do all it can to keep the blood within these limits. For example, if you eat a lot of acid-forming foods and have high stress in your life (which promotes acid) your body will store some of the acids in your tissues, rob some calcium (which is alkaline) from your bones and secrete acid through the kidneys in order to keep the blood at the correct pH. So to protect your skin tissues and kidneys from damage, and your bones from calcium loss it pays to have plenty of alkalising foods in your diet, and fewer — or a balance — of the acidifying ones.

Over the long term a diet rich in highly acid-forming foods (beef, corn, white flour and white sugar to name a few) will cause, among other issues, low-grade metabolic acidosis, which causes a decline in kidney function as you age, and loss of bone density. Keeping your diet in acid–alkaline balance (a balance of alkalising vegetables and healthy acid-forming foods such as fish, beans and wholegrains) promotes strong bones and lightens the acid burden your kidneys have to deal with each day. Alkalising foods also promote younger skin as they aid the removal of toxins from the body. When enough alkalising foods are consumed in the diet, the urine pH can exceed an alkaline reading of 7.5 and alkalisation occurs – this enhances the liver's ability to detoxify chemicals including preservatives, amines, food colourings, MSG and salicylates. For example, when the urine pH exceeds 7.5, three times the amount of salicylates are deactivated and removed from the body via the urine. This is especially useful if you have salicylate and chemical sensitivities as it decreases the occurrence of negative reactions to foods over time thus allowing you to eat a more varied diet. *Alkalising foods also thin the blood so blood flow to the skin is improved*, giving your skin a healthy glow.

It's easy to check if your diet is acid–alkaline balanced as you can test the pH of your saliva or urine using litmus paper (such as Easy pH). The reading will change throughout the day depending on what you eat and drink, and stress can also greatly increase acid in the body, so remember to relax and take care of your mental health too.

There is much debate as to what foods are alkalising and often most fruits and some grains are listed as alkalising, which is untrue — most fruits and all grains are acid-forming but you can still enjoy them when balanced with alkalising foods. Foods that are alkalising include raw almonds, pretty much all vegetables (not cooked spinach, but raw spinach is highly alkalising) and a few fruits including lemons, limes, avocado, raw tomato and bananas which are listed on the charts on pages 226–227. The recipes in this book show you how to prepare and serve tasty acid-alkaline balanced meals.

12. Kumato

Kumato, a sweet and semi-black tomato, possesses an important skin nutrient that regular tomatoes don't — it's rich in AGE-reducing anthocyanins, hence the blackened appearance of the skin. Kumatoes are also rich in vitamin C and beta-carotene, which are known to fight some forms of cancer and heart disease.

Like traditional tomatoes, Kumato tomatoes are rich in lycopene, an important red carotenoid. Lycopene builds up in the skin in direct proportion to how much lycopene is in your diet and has a mild sunscreen effect within the skin. Lycopene also helps the body remove toxins and carcinogens (cancer-causing substances) as it enhances phase I and II liver detoxification reactions, and it has anti-cancer and antioxidant properties.[33] Raw tomato is a rich source of lycopene but after cooking the lycopene content markedly increases. Tomatoes are a rich source of flavonoids including quercetin, which has strong anti-inflammatory and antioxidant properties that are wonderful for the skin.[34]

If you can't find Kumatoes look for Black Russian tomatoes or favour roma (plum), vine-ripened or grape tomatoes. Recipes include Guava and Rocket Salad (p. 188), Mango and Black Sesame Salad (p. 205) and Oregano Chicken Sticks (p. 208).

The top 12 anti-AGE foods can help you create younger skin and a healthy body, and the menus, beginning on p. 139, will show you how to incorporate them into your daily diet.

A quick recap

❋ Eat 1 cup of purple foods each day — such as purple salad leaves, purple kale, blueberries, red onion, red cabbage, eggplant (aubergine), purple broccoli or purple carrots — to encourage collagen production and reduce AGE formation.

❋ Eat ½ cup of red foods daily, including red quinoa, tomato, red capsicum (pepper), pomegranate and guava — this is important to ensure you consume enough vitamin C for collagen production.

❋ Eat a serve of black foods several times a week, such as 1 teaspoon of black sesame seeds or ½ cup of black quinoa or black rice, or a handful of Kumatoes or blackberries. Note that some black foods are not black due to anthocyanins — for example, black pasta is dyed with squid ink and does not contain anthocyanins.

❋ Add spices to your daily diet such as 1 tablespoon of yellow curry powder to make curries; make black tea special by adding a slice of fresh ginger and a clove; and control blood sugar with a small sprinkle of cinnamon on oats or added to smoothies, curries and casseroles.

❋ Use fresh lemon and lime in your cooking as they reduce AGE formation and supply vitamin C for collagen support.

Chapter 5

Other useful ingredients

Variety is not only the spice of life, it can help you to look younger for longer. It's important to eat a wide variety of healthy foods so the 28-day program also includes the following foods which are low in dietary AGEs and rich in nutrients, protein or dietary fibre for a balanced diet that's beneficial for the whole body.

Dark leafy greens

Dark green salad leaves are highly alkalising and beneficial for the skin thanks to their rich chlorophyll content. Dark leafy greens also deliver more nutrients for fewer calories and the calcium in kale and watercress is easy for the body to absorb. Greens contain antioxidants, folic acid, magnesium, calcium, beta-carotene, vitamin C, B-group vitamins, potassium and cancer-protective phyto-nutrients, plus they're gluten-free and low GI. Varieties include Chinese greens, kale, dandelion greens, silver beet, spinach, chicory, beet greens, mustard greens, rocket (arugula), watercress and baby spinach. Recipes include Green Glow Juice (p. 162), Scrambled Eggs with Watercress (p. 174), Guava and Rocket Salad (p. 188) and Watercress Soup (p. 182).

Liquid chlorophyll

Chlorophyll is the green pigment found in plants and it absorbs sunlight and converts it into plant energy. Chlorophyll is highly alkalising, it contains potassium and iron, and is rich in magnesium needed for cardiovascular and skin health. Chlorophyll increases oxygen-carrying capacity in the blood, which can give you more energy and stamina, and it has a blood-thinning effect which gives the skin a healthy glow. It promotes friendly bacteria in the bowel so it can reduce harmful bowel microbes; promotes healthy digestion; and prevents bad breath and body odour.

If you don't think you are getting enough greens in your diet, there are liquid chlorophyll supplements available which are excellent for skin health (available at health food shops and online). Just mix a teaspoon or two in a glass of water. Please note that using liquid chlorophyll is optional.

Apple cider vinegar

Vinegar has been used for medicinal purposes and to flavour and preserve foods for more than 2000 years.[1] Today apple cider vinegar (ACV) is the therapeutic vinegar of choice because it is strongly alkalising once digested (making it beneficial for the skin and the body's acid–alkaline balance). All other vinegars are strongly acidifying and are not recommended on a skin health program (but other vinegars can be enjoyed in moderation as a part of a healthy diet after the 28-day program).

According to studies, apple cider vinegar has the added benefits of lowering blood sugar and delaying gastric emptying, so it can be beneficial for reducing glycation.[2] Apple cider vinegar can be added to broths to help prevent AGE formation (Anti-ageing Broth on p. 176) or use apple cider vinegar to make salad dressings, such as Halo Dressing on p. 154 (with frequent use, this dressing on salads gives the skin a healthy glow).

Note: vinegar is strongly acidic before digestion so it must be diluted with water or put into a dressing or with other ingredients. Do not consume ACV without diluting it first and do not consume vinegar if you have gastric ulcers or sulfate sensitivity.

Grains

Grains supply dietary fibre which is essential for good bowel health and beautiful, blemish-free skin. Suitable flours and grains include spelt, rye, barley, quinoa, oats and oat bran. Favour wholegrains that have a low to medium GI rating. Basmati rice, Doongara rice and sushi rice are okay as they have a medium to low GI but other rice varieties are high GI. Most brown rice varieties have a high glycemic index, so favour brown rice labelled 'low GI' which is now available in some larger supermarkets. Avoid white bread, wheat flours, Turkish flat bread and puffed amaranth as the glycaemic index is incredibly high.

Spelt

Spelt is similar to wheat but it's easier to digest because of its lower gluten content — so you're less likely to bloat after eating it (which can mean a flatter stomach). Spelt flour is a popular wheat flour alternative, especially for those intolerant to wheat. It bakes beautifully when used in cooking (almost rising as much as wheat) and it tastes remarkably similar to wheat.

Spelt sourdough bread uses the traditional, non-yeast method of breadmaking, so it is naturally lower in phytic acid and it's low GI — good news for keeping blood sugar levels steady so there is less risk of AGE formation. If you can't find spelt sourdough bread or spelt tortillas or wraps in your local area you can bake your own flat bread — it's easy (see Spelt Flat Bread, p. 192). If you are gluten intolerant stick with gluten-free alternatives but first check if they're healthy, low GI and free of artificial additives.

Oats

Rolled or traditional oats make a fantastic low-AGE breakfast. Oats are a cereal grain containing small amounts of gluten. They are rolled flat, and this is how you want to buy them — not the ones which have been processed into instant oats as the extra processing gives them a higher GI so they can spike blood sugar levels, which is bad news for the skin.

Just your regular home-brand rolled oats (which are super cheap) will do. I recommend soaking them overnight to make the nutrients more available and cooking time quicker or, for younger skin, to make a delicious non-toasted raw muesli recipe called Omega Muesli (p. 169). If you are allergic to gluten or oats try the Quinoa Porridge recipe for breakfast (p. 171).

Tip: whenever consuming grains add a dash of ground cinnamon to keep your blood sugar levels from spiking too much.

Oils

For 28 days minimise cooking with oils, which are a rich source of AGEs. However, there are a couple of oils that are okay to use in moderation or raw in salads. Extra virgin olive oil that is *first cold pressed* may be used in salads and uncooked. The second option is rice bran oil that has been *extra cold filtered* — just check the label when purchasing. Rice bran oil has one of the highest smoke points, making it okay for cooking at moderate temperatures *if you must cook with oil.*

Smoke points of common cooking oils

Cooking oil	Smoking point °C	Smoking point °F
refined safflower oil	266°C	510°F
rice bran oil	254°C	490°F
ghee (Indian clarified butter)	252°C	485°F
refined/light olive oil	242°C	468°F
refined soybean oil	238°C	460°F
refined coconut oil	232°C	450°F
refined canola oil	204°C	400°F
extra virgin olive oil	190°C	375°F
extra virgin coconut oil	177°C	350°F
butter	121–149°C	250–300°F
virgin safflower oil	107°C	225°F

Protein foods

Here are some guidelines for choosing quality protein foods such as meats, eggs, fish and beans. Importantly, *protein from animal sources should be free range or organic where possible.* Avoid red meat for 28 days; if you like eating meat, favour skinless chicken, turkey, fish and seafood. Skinless chicken or turkey can be eaten once or twice a week and seafood one to three times a week, and then on the other days eat vegetarian options such as soups. (See menus, starting on p. 139, for more details.) Some other things to note:

- It's essential to remove chicken skin and cut off fatty pieces (the skin is incredibly rich in AGEs).
- Buy only the freshest cuts of meat which are free of preservatives and low in fat.
- If you are vegetarian favour eggs, tofu, beans and other legumes.
- Avoid vegetarian or vegan patties and meatless sausages, which contain artificial additives and/or require frying.
- If you are vegan make sure you eat legumes with a grain twice a day so you are consuming enough protein for healthy skin. For example, kidney beans or green beans or raw tofu served with rice or spelt pasta (plus vegies, of course).

Choose from the following animal and vegetable protein sources:

- chicken
- turkey
- fish and seafood (see p. 68)
- legumes (see p. 69)
- raw tofu
- green beans and peas
- eggs* (scrambled, boiled or poached)
- sprouts (bean, mung bean, lentil, pea, etc).

*Avoid eating raw egg whites as they can cause what is known as 'egg white injury', a biotin deficiency that causes skin rashes and other skin problems if raw eggs are eaten on a frequent basis.

Seafood

Studies show two to three serves of fish each week are beneficial for elevating mood and increasing the health of the brain, skin and heart — these benefits mainly come from the omega-3, EPA and DHA found in seafood, particularly in oily fish. Good sources of these nutrients include trout, salmon, sardines, herring and fish oil supplements. Other minor sources of EPA and DHA include low fat seafood such as carp, pike, haddock, oysters, clams, scallops and squid.

It's important to favour seafoods which are *low in mercury* as this heavy metal can be harmful to unborn babies, young children and during pregnancy, and it can also affect mental function and cause skin rashes. The general rule is: the higher up the food chain and the bigger the fish (e.g. shark/flake), the more mercury it could contain. There are plenty of low mercury choices, such as those listed below. If in doubt ask your local fishmonger.

Best seafood choices:

- trout and rainbow trout
- flathead
- dory (small fillets)
- hake
- bream
- shrimp
- flounder
- herring
- sardines
- lobster
- oysters
- quality canned tuna in springwater/brine*
- salmon
- other small fish.

*You can make a healthy snack with 85g (3oz) of canned tuna twice a week, as canned tuna is sourced from smaller-sized tuna.

Fish to avoid

The following fish contain high levels of mercury and should be avoided as often as possible:

- flake/shark (often used for fish and chips)
- large snapper
- swordfish
- marlin
- king mackerel
- perch (orange roughy)
- barramundi (larger fish)
- gemfish
- ling
- larger-sized tuna (e.g. albacore, southern blue fin).

Australian health authorities recommend if you eat a serve of mercury-rich fish you should then avoid eating all seafood for at least 2 weeks afterwards to allow time for your mercury levels to reduce.

Legumes

Legumes are rich in magnesium and potassium and supply dietary fibre, protein and slow-release carbohydrate for energy. Canned legumes such as brown lentils, chickpeas (garbanzo beans) and mixed beans are a convenient option but I recommend cooking them fresh as the canned varieties may contain bisphenol A (BPA) — a substance used to coat the cans. The Food Standards Agency in the United Kingdom says that BPA is known to have 'weak oestrogenic effects' and it could disrupt hormone systems. Dried legumes which are home-cooked are the best and most nutritious choice.

Cooking guide for legumes
Step 1: Rinsing

Rinse the legumes and pick out any discoloured or shrivelled legumes or small stones.

Step 2: Soaking

Soak the dried legumes to reduce phytic acid, promote even cooking and reduce simmering time. Bring a large saucepan of water to the boil then add the legumes and boil for 2 minutes. Remove from heat, cover and soak overnight. After soaking, discard the soaked water as it contains the indigestible sugars that promote gas.

Step 3: Cooking

After soaking the legumes (if required), add 4 cups of water for every 1 cup of legumes. Place into a medium-sized saucepan, cover with a lid and bring to the boil. Reduce to a simmer and check often. Avoid stirring the beans while cooking and do not add salt as it can toughen the beans if added too early.

Lentils are quick to cook, but for all other beans check their progress after 45 minutes – if the legumes are cooked they should be soft enough to easily mash using the back of a fork. All cooking times are approximate and will vary depending on how long it has been since the legumes were harvested.

Legume cooking times

Legume	Approximate cooking times
adzuki beans	45 minutes–1½ hours
black-eyed peas/beans	1–2 hours
cannellini (white) beans	1 hour
chickpeas (garbanzo beans)	1½–2 hours (allow to cool in cooking water)
dried split peas	up to 45 minutes
kidney beans	1 hour+
lentils	20–30 minutes
lima beans	1–2 hours
mung beans	45–60 minutes
navy beans	1–2 hours
pinto beans	1–2 hours

What types of dried legumes do not need soaking?

Dried lentils (red and brown/green), split peas (green and yellow) and black-eyed peas do not need to be soaked but you can soak them if you suffer from poor digestion. Adzuki and mung beans only need to be soaked for 1 to 2 hours. However, make sure you rinse these beans and lentils thoroughly, changing the water two or three times until it runs clear.

Rice malt syrup

Ideally, your diet should have no added sweeteners, but for those of you who wish to use sweetener the best choice is rice malt syrup for two reasons: it is alkalising (whereas all other sweeteners convert to acid in the body) and very mild in flavour so it does not cause sugar cravings. It can be found in most health food shops and some larger supermarkets stock brands such as Pureharvest.

Sea salt

Commercial table salt usually has added anti-caking agent with aluminium, most of the nutritious minerals have been removed and it's acid-producing so it can disrupt the body's acid–alkaline balance if used frequently. For these reasons it is best to avoid consuming commercial table salt (you can, however, add it to your clothes wash to colour-fast dark clothes).

If you would like to use salt on your meals buy quality sea salt such as Celtic or macro sea salt — the best salts are grey in colour, indicating minimal processing and maximum mineral content. Quality sea salt may also be slightly damp or chunky if there is no anti-caking agent. These alkaline salts are okay to use in moderation, however, do not add salt to your food if you have high blood pressure.

Non-dairy milks

Dairy products, especially animal milks (including cow, goat and sheep milk), can contribute to excessively dry and prematurely aged skin and oily skin conditions such as acne. Through my years of working with eczema sufferers and people with severe skin disorders I have found that most skin problems can be improved by avoiding cow's milk and other dairy products, along with an increase in alkalising foods in the diet.

According to an article published in the *Harvard University Gazette*, dairy products are rich in animal sex hormones and pregnant cows are commonly milked in Western countries with their milk containing up to 33 times more oestrogen than milk from a non-pregnant cow.[3] A single cow provides almost 200,000 glasses of milk in her lifetime! The scientists from the Harvard School of Public Health went on to say that butter, milk and cheese are implicated in higher rates of hormone-dependent cancers in humans, although more research is needed.

This is a dairy-free program and there are a couple of suitable milk alternatives to choose from for those of you who would like to consume non-dairy milk in your porridge, tea, coffee, smoothies or baked goods.

Organic soy milk

Unlike dairy milks, which are often rich in fats, lactose and cholesterol, soy milk is low in saturated fat, lactose-free and can help to lower cholesterol and protect blood vessels from damage. Soy milk contains fewer sugars and calories than regular cow's milk, which has around 12g (⅖oz) of sugar per cup (as it's rich in lactose, a milk sugar) and in comparison soy milk has less than 6g (⅕oz) per cup.

Soy milk contains phytoestrogens or 'plant oestrogens' that are weaker than human or animal hormones. Research shows these phytoestrogens can be beneficial for people with low oestrogen levels or those who are going through menopause. Phytoestrogens can promote calcium absorption in your body and this can reduce the risk of bone fractures and osteoporosis.

Like all processed food products, soy milk has its good and not-so-good points and there are different qualities available. The best choice is soy milk containing *organic whole soybeans* as these are less processed and of the highest quality. Also choose one with added calcium, for bone health. Avoid soy milk listing *soy isolate* as an ingredient, as soy isolate was once considered a waste product and may contain aluminium. Furthermore, if you use soy milk made with whole soybeans you're getting better (complete, or whole) protein, whereas soy milk made with isolate isn't a good protein source. If you have unusually high levels of oestrogen in your body then soy milk may not be suitable for you; if you are concerned, your doctor can check your oestrogen levels or just try delicious almond milk instead, or rice milk if you don't like almond milk (keep in mind that rice milk has a high GI so you will need to add cinnamon to it).

FAQ: 'Can people with gluten intolerance drink soy milk?'

Yes, but you need to buy a specific type. The ingredient *barley malt*, which is added to most soy milks, contains gluten so if you are gluten intolerant look for *malt-free soy milk* or choose almond milk instead.

Almond milk

Historically, almond milk was popular in medieval Europe and throughout the Middle East. Today it is gaining popularity once again as a high protein alternative to regular cow's milk. Almonds supply vitamin E, magnesium, selenium, zinc, potassium and calcium, and a range of antioxidants which can slow or inhibit AGE formation. Unlike cow's milk, which contains cholesterol, almond milk is cholesterol-free and has a cholesterol-lowering effect thanks to its flavonoid content.

Almond milk has a moisture-boosting effect on the skin so if you have dry skin this milk is for you (however, if you have oily skin and breakouts occur after you change to almond milk then discontinue use). If you have acne or oily skin then organic soy milk would be your best choice. Almond milk is available at health food shops and many supermarkets but it's also super easy to make; the recipe is on p. 168. Use the leftover almond meal as a body scrub to gently exfoliate your skin.

Linseeds/flaxseeds

Linseeds, also known as flaxseeds, are small brown seeds best known for their rich content of anti-inflammatory omega-3. The seeds are a source of phytochemicals, silica, mucilage, oleic acid, protein, vitamin E and dietary fibre, for gastrointestinal and liver health. Flaxseed oil contains more than 50 per cent omega-3 essential fatty acids and it's beneficial for dry skin conditions.

To demonstrate how essential fatty acids influence the skin, scientists gave two groups of women either flaxseed or borage oil — both rich sources of omega-3 and containing smaller amounts of omega-6 — for 12 weeks and a third group received a placebo, which was olive oil. After 6 weeks of consuming only 1 teaspoon of either flaxseed oil or borage oil per day, skin water loss was decreased by about 10 per cent, and by week 12 the flaxseed oil group showed further protection from water loss and the skin was significantly more hydrated. While the olive oil (placebo) group showed no significant change in skin health, at 12 weeks the flaxseed oil group had significantly less skin reddening, roughness and scaling.[4] Flaxseeds can also accelerate wound healing and reduce inflammation and all-round skin sensitivity.[5,6] Due to its moisture-boosting effect, flaxseed oil and linseeds may not be suitable if you are prone to breakouts or have oily skin.

Linseed/flaxseed daily intake

Adults with dry and ageing skin can have 2–4 teaspoons of whole linseeds daily or 2 teaspoons of flaxseed oil to boost skin moisture and promote smoother skin. Drink plenty of water when eating linseeds as the fibre absorbs about five times the seeds' weight.

Storage tips for flaxseed oil and flaxseeds

Omega-3 is highly unstable so it's easily damaged by heat and once linseeds/flaxseeds have been processed into oil or ground into a fine powder they can go rancid within several weeks especially if not stored correctly. For these reasons do not buy pre-ground linseeds/flaxseeds or LSA (a ground mix containing linseeds, sunflower seeds and almonds). Whole linseeds are the best way to consume this super seed.

If buying flaxseed oil, it must be refrigerated practically at all times. Flaxseed oil must not be heated or used for frying, and used up within 4 or 5 weeks. *Whole flaxseeds/linseeds are easy to keep fresh*, they are quite heat resistant but store them in the refrigerator to increase shelf life. They're great in smoothies (see p. 164), or try Flaxseed Lemon Drink (p. 165) and Omega Muesli (p. 169).

FAQ: 'Can I eat chia seeds as they're also rich in omega-3?'

Chia seeds have only recently become popular so there is not a lot of scientific research on the health benefits of this tiny seed. However, what we do know is they are a rich source of omega-3 (with more than 50 per cent omega-3) so they can be a nutritious alternative to linseeds/flaxseeds.

Chapter 6

Anti-AGE supplements

As you age, your skin becomes drier, nutrient levels decline and wrinkle formation is accelerated. Extra assistance through supplementation can help to slow some biochemical changes that occur with ageing and boost skin moisture so your skin appears more youthful. Here are the top 5.

Health note

Before taking supplements of any kind, seek advice from your doctor, especially if you are taking medical drugs, are pregnant or breastfeeding as the following supplements can have a detox effect and may not be suitable for you. Some supplements such as omega-3 and vitamin C thin the blood so avoid these supplements if you are on blood-thinning or heart medications or preparing for surgery, laser treatments, injections or childbirth. There are food alternatives for most supplements so you can do this program without supplements if required.

1. Calcium

You may know that calcium is good for your bones and for calming the nervous system so you have a good night's sleep, but what you may not realise is how important calcium is for your skin, especially the upper layer. Calcium promotes a healthy acid mantle, which protects your skin from microbe invasion and infections. The epidermis layer of the skin must also respond to weather extremes and calcium helps to maintain the right amount of moisturising lipids by triggering their production in low humidity or when required. These lipids are water-resistant so they trap water in the skin so it does not dry out.

Low calcium levels in the epidermis hamper the skin's natural exfoliating process so dead skin cells build up and this leads to greater premature ageing and skin that appears dry and dull.

The research ...

* In healthy skin, high concentrations of calcium and magnesium are present in the upper epidermis.[1]
* If the moisture level in the air drops, calcium triggers the skin to increase the production of lipids and the epidermis thickens in order to trap moisture in your skin.[2]
* According to research, intake of calcium, retinol and the collagen-promoting nutrients vitamin C, magnesium, iron and zinc appear to be protective against UV-induced skin ageing.[3]

The calcium paradox is that dairy products, which are rich in calcium, can contribute to skin problems including acne, eczema and cellulite (possibly due to the presence of animal hormones and high AGEs and the absence of the right supporting nutrients), while calcium in supplement form has a youth-promoting effect on ageing skin. Calcium, when taken with a healthy diet and with magnesium, vitamin D and collagen-supporting nutrients zinc, manganese and copper, helps to tighten up connective tissue and reduces the appearance of cellulite and sagging skin within 28 days.

Dosage information

Dosage for adults: 1000 to 1200mg of calcium daily in divided doses, taken in between meals so it does not interfere with the absorption of other minerals. If you are post-menopausal, pregnant, breastfeeding or have poor bone density take 1200mg daily. Ideally choose a calcium supplement that contains a combination of calcium citrate (avoid calcium carbonate), vitamin D, magnesium, zinc, manganese and copper (see 'Resources', p. 233).

Caution: Calcium supplementation can interfere with drug absorption so speak with your doctor before taking calcium if you are on medication or are unwell. Do not take antacids containing aluminium while taking calcium.

2. Vitamin C

The body is truly remarkable and resourceful. It makes many of its own vitamins in the gastrointestinal tract and it stores minerals in the liver and bones; however, the body does not store or manufacture vitamin C so it must be consumed in your diet every day. Vitamin C (also known as ascorbic acid) aids the absorption of iron and copper, boosts the formation of collagen in the skin, guards against infections and is required for liver detoxification. Vitamin C also inhibits glycation and AGE formation so it's an important anti-ageing nutrient.[4]

Vitamin C is a natural antihistamine as it destroys the imidazole ring of the histamine molecule. For this reason it's imperative that allergy sufferers avoid developing vitamin C deficiency as it can result in histamine toxicity and allergic reactions may increase in severity. You need to consume at least 45mg of vitamin C every day to avoid developing deficiency signs but higher amounts are needed to reduce the severity of allergies, boost collagen production in the skin and for optimal health. See p. 90 for vitamin C deficiency symptoms.

Food sources of vitamin C

Food sources (100g/3½ oz)	Vitamin C content in milligrams per 100g
guava	245mg
red capsicum (pepper)	170mg
brussels sprouts	110mg
broccoli	105mg
green capsicum (pepper)	90mg
cauliflower	70mg
pawpaw	60mg
strawberries (1 cup)	55mg
lemon (1 medium)	50mg
sweet potato	30mg
white potato (1 medium)	30mg

Dosage information

Dosage for adults: consume between 50 to 200mg of vitamin C daily *from foods* — the menus will help you do this. As ascorbic acid (the general form of vitamin C) is acidic, if buying a supplement look for *buffered* vitamin C, which has an alkaline mineral added to it such as magnesium ascorbate, potassium ascorbate, sodium ascorbate or calcium ascorbate.

Caution: Vitamin C thins the blood. Do not take vitamin C supplements if you have haemochromatosis or if you have been prescribed aspirin, anticoagulants or antidepressants. See 'Health note' on p. 77.

3. Chromium

The mineral chromium is required in micro amounts for normal growth and general health, and it's needed for the breakdown of proteins, carbohydrates and fats. It's the active ingredient in 'glucose tolerance factor' and it enhances the action of the hormone insulin, which helps your body control glucose in the blood. Chromium's action of *helping the body to correctly process glucose (blood sugar) for energy use* reduces the risk of advanced glycation end products and protects collagen from irreparable damage. It can also dampen sugar cravings. Deficiency symptoms are listed on p. 90.

Food sources of chromium

Food sources	Chromium content in micrograms per 100g
2 cups cos (romaine) lettuce	15.6mcg
½ cup raw onion	12.4mcg
100g (3½oz) turkey meat	10.4mcg
1 cup cooked peas	6mcg
1 teaspoon dried garlic	3mcg
1 cup mashed potato	3mcg
2 slices wholemeal bread	2mcg
1 medium banana	1mcg
½ cup green beans	1mcg

Dosage information

Dosage for adults: 45–60mcg (ug) elemental chromium daily from foods and supplement. It is ideal to have a chromium supplement in divided doses with each main meal. Note: mcg is also written as ug.

Caution: If you are taking medical drugs, consult with a nutritionist or doctor before taking chromium. If you have insulin-dependent diabetes seek advice from your doctor before supplementing with chromium as it alters blood sugar levels (insulin would need to be reduced if you were taking chromium but do this *only* with your doctor's supervision).

While statistics on chromium deficiency are limited, data from research suggests that only 0.4–2.5 per cent of chromium is absorbed from foods. Vitamin C and vitamin B3 (niacin) enhance the absorption of chromium, as does protein, so take a chromium supplement with a protein-rich meal. Chromium picolinate is easier for the body to absorb than other types of chromium and a chromium supplement should also contain vitamins B3, B6, B12, vitamin C, vitamin D3, folic acid, magnesium and zinc.

4. Essential fatty acids

Essential fatty acids (EFAs) are vital for healthy skin and are classified as 'essential' because your body cannot manufacture them and they must be obtained from your diet. The two main groups of essential fatty acids are omega-3 and omega-6. Omega-6 is present in vegetable oils, margarine, nuts and seeds and is usually over-consumed in the Western diet (which can lead to oily skin and blemishes if you are prone to these conditions).

Rich sources of omega-3 include linseeds/flaxseeds, chia seeds, fresh walnuts and fish, especially trout, salmon and sardines. Omega-3 works to create younger skin a number of ways. It converts to potent anti-inflammatory substances called EPA (eicosapentaenoic acid) and DHA (docosahexaenoic acid), which are omega-3 in its more potent form. EPA and DHA calm skin inflammation, reduce skin sensitivity and enhance the immune system (they're great for the heart too).

Balancing the fats in your diet

Both omega-6 and omega-3 make a noticeable difference to oil production and the moisture content of the skin but you should consume them in a 1:1 ratio (in typical Western diets the ratio is more like 20:1). To amend the ratios of these fats in your diet, eat fewer processed vegetable oils (and fewer fatty meats), ditch margarine and add fish, seafood and/or flaxseeds/linseeds into your diet. If you are vegetarian or vegan, favour fresh walnuts, flaxseeds or chia seeds. Dark leafy greens also contain small amounts of omega-3.

Food sources of omega-3

Food (standard serve)	omega-3 content in milligrams
salmon, 113g (4oz)	2000mg
linseeds/flaxseeds, 3 teaspoons	1750mg
2 x omega-3 fortified eggs	1114mg
scallops, 113g (4oz)	1100mg
halibut, baked, 113g (4oz)	620mg

Food sources of EPA and DHA

(these are the active/therapeutic compounds within omega-3)

Food: 100g (3½oz) unless specified	EPA/DHA in milligrams
Atlantic salmon	1090–1830mg*
fresh tuna	240–1280mg*
herring	1710–1810mg*
sardines	980–1700mg*
rainbow trout	840–980mg*
mackerel	340–1570mg*
canned tuna in water, drained	260–730mg*
flaxseed oil, 3 teaspoons (15ml/½fl oz)	850mg
flaxseeds/linseeds, ground or whole, 3 teaspoons	220mg

*The EPA and DHA content varies depending on whether the skin has been left on or removed: fish with skin on is higher in fat so it is a richer source of omega-3 fatty acids, EPA and DHA.

Dosage information

To avoid deficiency, your EPA/DHA dosage should be at least 600mg per day. Adults who want to treat very dry skin, wrinkles and premature ageing can take up to 2000mg EPA/DHA per day* in divided doses (approximately 6g of omega-3 depending on brand but lower doses may also be effective).

*On the days you eat fresh fish or seafood you can skip taking an omega-3 supplement. If you do not want to take fish oil supplements or eat fish, just add flaxseeds/linseeds and flaxseed oil into your diet (see p. 74).

Caution: Omega-3 has many benefits but supplements are not suitable for everyone. Do not take flaxseed oil or high-dose omega-3 oils if you have acne or are prone to breakouts, as doing so may increase skin oiliness. Check 'Health note' on p. 77 to see if this supplement is right for you.

5. Carotenoids

Research shows that eating foods rich in cryptoxanthin, a carotenoid that supplies vitamin A, significantly boosts skin hydration.[5] Carotenoids, such as beta-carotene and cryptoxanthin, are potent AGE inhibitors and should be consumed daily but preferably not in supplement form as they work best when packaged in fresh fruits and vegetables.

Cryptoxanthin-rich foods include papaya, pawpaw, pumpkin (winter squash), paprika, persimmons, capsicum (peppers) and peaches. Beta-carotene-rich foods include carrots, beetroot and sweet potato.

Dosage information

Have at least one serve of carotenoid-rich fruit or vegetables daily — at least half a cup. Recipes include Peach, Thyme and Chilli Marinade (p. 150), Papaya Cups with Lime and Guava (p. 159), Mediterranean Seafood Soup (p. 206), Spiced Sweet Potato Soup (p. 175) and Sweet Potato Salad (p. 200).

Nutrients for collagen production

If you were to build a house you would ideally use a supply of strong, weather-resistant materials such as timber, concrete, nails, bricks and so on. Then as the years passed by, you would repair any breakages, give it a new coat of paint and if the roof leaked you would maybe replace a few tiles and fix the guttering. It's a similar story with your skin: you need to supply the right building materials from your diet so your body can make healthy skin, then you need a constant supply of the right nutrients for maintenance, repair and renewing of skin cells and collagen.

Collagen is like the glue that holds your skin firmly in place and gives it resilience. But collagen does not magically appear or stay the same once it's formed. More than one third of collagen is made up of the amino acid glycine, another third is proline and the rest consists of lysine and other amino acids, supplied by protein-containing foods such as fish, eggs, meats, beans, nuts and seeds. Lysine and proline need co-factors vitamin C, iron and manganese to form strong collagen in the skin, and zinc is vital for collagen formation.

If your diet lacked even just one of the right collagen-building nutrients it would be like holidaying in a house made of straw or bamboo — it might look like a Balinese resort online but in reality it's a building that leaks whenever it rains and there is never a repairman when you need one. Your diet might consist of the most decadent foods (see 'The prisoner study' following) but without the right nutrients to aid the structural formation of collagen, the skin, tendons and blood vessels become fragile, your skin can also become over-sensitive to its environment (the weather, skin products and pollen to name a few) and skin ageing is accelerated. The following scientific study published in the *American Journal of Clinical Nutrition* illustrates this perfectly.[6] (This study was conducted in the days before the ethical implications of conducting experiments on prisoners were a consideration.)

The prisoner study

In 1969, six prisoners were involved in a scientific diet experiment which involved eating pancakes, bacon, cooked egg whites, noodles and butterscotch pudding with marshmallows and meringue. They also ate chocolate, candy, muffins, seafood, chicken casseroles and gingerbread cookies and drank strawberry-flavoured soft drink (a diet similar to what some children and Western families eat today). However, vitamin C was missing from the diet and to ensure it was the only deficiency the prisoners suffered from (as this diet could have given them a few malnutrition problems), they were given a vitamin and mineral supplement that supplied everything except for vitamin C.

After 3 weeks of being on this decadent diet the scientists reported the prisoners' gums started to swell and bleed and their skin developed small bumps, which worsened over time. Several men developed infections including sore throat, ear infection and fevers. Two of the inmates escaped at this point. The rest of the prisoners continued with the diet until their skin literally began to fall apart. On day 36 of the diet, one prisoner had to have two teeth removed and the prisoners complained of fatigue and muscle cramps. On the 52nd day mild haemorrhaging of the skin and follicles occurred, blood began spotting in the eyes and skin bumpiness increased as collagen could no longer form properly without vitamin C. The study was halted at this point.[7]

Nutrients for collagen formation

Here is a list of the nutrients your body absolutely needs to build strong and healthy collagen and *they can all be obtained through your diet*, along with the supplement routine detailed in the Resources section of the book (p. 233).

Nutrient for collagen formation + daily intake	Food sources — nutrient content in mg per 100g/3½oz (unless specified)
Protein (supplies amino acids such as glycine, proline and lysine) AI: 1g of protein per 1kg of body weight per day (more for athletes) RDI: 64g (2¼oz) for men; 46g (1½oz) for women; 65g (2¼oz) if pregnant or breastfeeding	150g (5oz) cooked chicken (42g/½oz) 150g (5oz) cooked fish (36g/11/3oz) canned tuna or salmon (24g/¾oz) 1 cup cooked legumes (16g/½oz) 6 king prawns (14g/½oz) 1 egg (6g¼oz)
Glycine (one-third of collagen is made up of this amino acid; protein foods are rich in glycine) Recommended intake: 2–5g	Richest sources are: broth (Anti-ageing Broth, p. 176) and unsweetened gelatine powder (10g/½oz contains 1904mg) raw soybeans (1880mg) turkey or chicken with skin (1395mg) split peas (1092mg) crab meat (1089mg) raw tuna (1056mg) buckwheat (1031mg) raw salmon (1022mg) red lentils (1014mg) rainbow trout (1002mg) 20g (2/3oz) linseeds (250mg)
Iron RDI: 9mg for men; 18mg for women	mussels (8mg) oysters (6mg) scallops (3mg) wholemeal bread (3mg) 1 cup cooked lentils (3.6mg) pepitas (green pumpkin seeds) (10mg) soy milk (7–9mg) tempeh (7.2mg) tofu (2.8mg) 1 tbs tahini (1.2mg) chicken (1mg)

Nutrient for collagen formation + daily intake	Food sources — nutrient content in mg per 100g/3½oz (unless specified)
Zinc AI: 8mg Recommended intake: 14–20mg	oysters (45mg) crab (4mg) wholemeal bread (8mg) canned sardines (5mg) brazil nuts (4mg) poached eggs (3.6mg) dried apricots (3.2mg) almonds (3mg) chicken (2mg) rolled oats (1.8mg) salmon (1mg) lentils (1mg)
Manganese AI: 2mg RDI: 2–5mg	spelt (1.87mg) 1 handful almonds (0.65mg) 1 cup cooked chickpeas (1.7mg) 1 cup cooked oats (1.3mg) 1 cup cooked lima beans (1.1mg) 1 oatbran muffin (1.5mcg) ½ cup brown rice (1.07mg) 1 cup mashed sweet potato (0.88mg) 1 cup green tea (1mg) 1 cup black tea (0.47mg)
Silicon (silica) Recommended intake: 10–25mg[8]	dried dates (16mg) (3 dates = 7mg) oat cereals/granola (12mg) porridge oats (11mg) wheatbran cereal (11mg) green beans or French (8.7mg) boiled fresh spinach (5mg) wholemeal bread (5mg) red lentils (4mg) oatbran (23mg) (2 tbs bran = 3mg)

Nutrient for collagen formation + daily intake	Food sources — nutrient content in mg per 100g/3½oz (unless specified)
Vitamin C AI: 45mg Recommended intake: 50–200mg	Refer to p. 80
Copper AI: 1.7mg Recommended intake: 2–3mg	oysters (7.6mg) crab (4.8mg) brazil nuts (1.1mg) wholemeal bread (0.8mg) prawns (0.7mg) mushrooms (0.6mg) spinach (0.3mg) sweet potato (0.2mg) salmon (0.1mg)

AI = adequate intake for adults to avoid deficiency

RDI = recommended daily intake as per Australian Government health guidelines

Recommended intake = my recommended daily intake for younger skin.

FAQ: 'How many supplements do I need to take for younger skin?'

Firstly read 'Health note' on p. 77 to check if supplementation is right for you. If you are okay to take supplements you can take the following:

1. Calcium supplement with added vitamin D (daily, taken before breakfast and dinner).

2. Chromium, with added vitamin C, B3, B6, magnesium, manganese and zinc (daily, taken with breakfast and lunch).

3. If you are a woman or vegetarian or vegan, take a herbal iron supplement daily to boost collagen production in the skin (see 'Resources' on p. 233 and iron information on p. 92).

Your diet should supply the other nutrients for healthy skin, and the menus and shopping list in Part 2 will make this easy for you. The only reasons to take an additional supplement would be if you have deficiency symptoms or if you have been prescribed a supplement for medical reasons. Do the following Nutrient Deficiency Questionnaire to see if you need to take additional supplements (or have a health check-up).

Nutrient Deficiency Questionnaire

What is your body trying to tell you?

We are often taught to accept ourselves the way we are, but what if your skin problems are trying to tell you something important about your health? Nutritional deficiencies accelerate skin ageing and cause a range of unpleasant symptoms which can worsen over time and lead to serious health complications if left untreated. Check if you have signs of nutritional deficiencies by circling any signs and symptoms you have in the following questionnaire. Please note the following symptoms can be caused by other factors and this questionnaire does not take the place of medical advice. An asterisk* denotes a symptom that you may need to discuss with your doctor in order to rule out other factors.

Vitamin C (ascorbic acid)

cravings for sweets or fruit
easy bruising or small purplish spots on skin*
swollen or bleeding gums
haemorrhaging*
frequent nosebleeds*
allergies*
dry skin
bumpy/rough skin or rash
poor wound healing*
frequent colds and flu
depression*
anaemia*
tooth loss*
fluid retention or swelling of lower limbs*
fatigue

Chromium

high blood sugar (pre-diabetes, type II diabetes)*
hypoglycaemia/low blood sugar
premature ageing
poor concentration*
irritability or dizziness after 2 to 6 hours without food*
need for frequent meals
cravings for sweets, carbs or alcohol
acne/pimples*
anxiety attacks*
excessive thirst*
ADD/ADHD*
depression*
fatigue in between meals

Copper
muscle disease*
age spots
sagging skin
impaired growth*
liver cancer*
loss of pigmentation
neurological symptoms*

Vitamin K
(deficiency is rare)
easy bruising
blood oozing from gums or nose*
excessive bleeding from cuts (slow to clot)*
osteoporosis*
easily fractured bones*

Vitamin B2 (riboflavin)
dermatitis
broken capillaries on face
sore, dry or cracked lips
mouth sores
red, sore tongue
sore or gritty feeling in eyes
oily or dull hair
increased sensitivity to light
split nails
loss of eyebrows/hair loss*

Vitamin B3 (niacin)
dermatitis
diarrhoea*
depression*
blood sugar problems
red, rough skin
pimples
low energy
muscular weakness*
bleeding gums*
cracked corners of mouth

Selenium
liver cancer*
muscle weakness and wasting*
inflammation or damaged heart muscles*
poor immunity
inability to cope with stress*

Silica
brittle fingernails
dry, brittle or thin hair
bone abnormalities*
joint problems*
premature ageing

Vitamin A and beta-carotene
acne
bumpy skin on backs of upper arms
poor night vision
scaly and dry skin
rough skin on heels
frequent colds or infections
dandruff
mouth ulcers
diarrhoea*
dry eyes

Vitamin B1 (thiamine)
burning feet
irritability
nervous conditions*
muscle atrophy*
loss of appetite*
pins and needles/numbness*
rapid heartbeat*
constipation*
poor circulation*
general weakness*

Vitamin B6 (pyridoxine)

acne

dermatitis

muscle weakness*

anaemia*

convulsions*

cracked skin at corners of mouth

mood changes/irritability

low blood sugar/hypoglycaemia

numbness or cramps in arms or legs*

smooth, painful tongue*

frequent colds or flu

Biotin (vitamin B7)

dermatitis or eczema

greyish skin colour or pallor*

dry skin

scaly lips

depression* or moodiness

premature greying of hair

red, scaly skin around eyes*

muscle pain*

dandruff

anxiety/inability to cope*

localised numbness*

loss of appetite*

Folic acid (vitamin B9)

anaemia*

shortness of breath*

pallor/pale complexion*

gastrointestinal disorders*

diarrhoea*

cracked lips and corners of mouth

inflamed tongue

depression*

irritability or hostility*

forgetfulness or sluggishness

insomnia*

Vitamin B12 (cobalamin)

anaemia*

fatigue

shortness of breath*

pallor/pasty complexion

nervousness or anxiety*

depression*

constipation*

red, smooth tongue

numb/tingling hands and feet*

poor coordination

dark, thin or spoon-shaped nails

Iodine

dry skin and hair

infertility*

miscarriages*

swollen neck (goitre)*

slow metabolism*

unexplained weight gain*

intolerance to cold weather

puffiness under eyes

depression*

constipation*

low sex drive*

Iron

anaemia*

pale palm creases

pale eyelid rims (should be pink)

pallor or greyish skin*

constipation*

spoon-shaped nails

ridges lengthwise in nails

split fingernails that won't heal

laboured breathing*

cravings for ice, clay or starch

dizziness*

sore tongue

heart palpitations*

Magnesium

cravings for alcohol or sugar

muscle twitching or weakness*

clicking joints

irregular heartbeat*

muscle cramps or pain*

tender calf muscles

soft or brittle nails

PMS

convulsions*

anxiety or irritability

insomnia*

Manganese

skin rash

abnormal blood sugar levels

impaired growth*

muscle twitching

growing pains during childhood

poor balance

convulsions*

bone malformations*

elevated blood calcium (test results)

weakness or dizziness*

iron-deficiency anaemia*

Calcium

muscle twitching*

cramps or aches*

stiff sore neck, ribcage pain, backache*

rickets, poor bone health*, osteoporosis*

cellulite and/or poor skin tone

insomnia*

numbness, tingling fingers*,
arms and/or legs*

lethargy

poor appetite*

dry skin

excessive irritability or nerves

Vitamin D

rickets/bowed legs*

bone deformities*

osteoporosis*

frequent backache*

eczema or psoriasis

fatigue

muscle weakness*

muscle twitching or spasms*

joint pain or stiffness*

Vitamin E (d-alpha-tocopherol)

(deficiency is rare)

dry skin

skin inflammation*

premature ageing*

loss of delicate sense of touch*

infertility*

miscarriages*

anaemia*

poor balance/equilibrium*

restless legs*

gluten intolerance*

abnormal eye movements*

frequent diarrhoea with fat in stools*

Essential fatty acids
(omega-3 and/or omega-6)

skin rashes

dry skin

dry, brittle hair or dandruff

bumps on the backs of upper arms

learning difficulties

hyperactivity, ADD/ADHD*

poor wound healing*

frequent infections

infertility*

arthritis*

depression*

weakness

poor vision

Molybdenum
sensitivity to sulfates and sulfur
sensitivity to chemicals
rapid heart rate*
rapid breathing*
headaches*
night blindness*

Potassium
hypokalemia*
fatigue*
muscle weakness and cramps*
tetany
intestinal paralysis*
bloating
constipation*
abdominal pain*
abnormal heartbeat*

Zinc
poor sense of taste or smell
acne or oily skin
stretch marks
white-coated tongue
white spots on fingernails
split, brittle or peeling fingernails
ridges on fingernails
anorexia or poor appetite*
diarrhoea*
impotence*
infertility*
frequent infections* or colds/flu
poor wound healing*
skin lesions*
frizzy hair or hair loss

Analysing the questionnaire

If you have three or more symptoms (per category) you may have a deficiency that requires supplementation or further investigation. However, a single unpleasant symptom can be an early warning sign that you have a mineral deficiency that needs attention. For example, if you have a split fingernail that won't heal you should investigate the cause — it could be something as simple as early iron-deficiency caused by drinking tea *during meals* as the tannins bind with iron from the meal, making it unavailable.

If you find you have *many* nutrient deficiencies it could indicate any of the following: digestive problems, malabsorption, candidiasis/fungal infestation, malnutrition, poor diet, excess alcohol consumption, early disease states or excess laxative use, to name a few.

Unpleasant symptoms are your body's way of saying 'look after me and investigate further'. If symptoms don't quickly improve with supplementation then it's important to speak with your doctor or health care professional for a formal diagnosis.

Chapter 7

Younger skin care

By choosing beauty products that contain *active* ingredients you can do more than moisturise your skin — you can create smoother skin, stimulate the production of new collagen, encourage faster cell renewal and make your skin look younger! The right skin care ingredients can also help to protect your skin from environmental damage and UV radiation. There are many, many skin care ingredients that are great for moisturising the skin (and I will cover these too) but this chapter focuses on the top 5 *active* skin care ingredients for creating younger skin. Then, there are some guidelines to choosing and using make-up to your best advantage.

FAQ: 'Do I need to change my skin care routine?'

If you already like your skin care routine and if you prefer to focus on your diet during the 28 days that is fine, just ensure your skin care products aren't causing breakouts or drying out your skin. If you are under 30 years old and already have good skin then you might not need to change your skin care routine but if you have sun-damaged skin then a bit of extra assistance can help you look years younger. Later in this chapter there are examples of skin care regimes for those who want to try something new.

FAQ: 'Do I begin a new skin care routine at the same time as changing my diet?'

Ideally you want to keep the two separate so you can see if a skin care product is right for you. If you drastically change your diet and start using new skin care products on the same day and your skin breaks out then it will be hard to tell if it is a reaction to the skin care product or if you are sensitive to a particular food or experiencing a typical detox symptom. It is recommended to start the new diet program at least a few days beforehand. You will probably need to take your time choosing the right skin care products for your skin type (and budget!), and testing the products in the store or asking for samples can help. Also, you may have to wait for products to be in stock or be sent to you if ordering online so this can delay the beginning of your skin care routine.

FAQ: 'What skin care products do you recommend?'

This is the question most often asked when people email me. While I do not endorse any particular products, in order to save you frustration I have mentioned a range of skin care brands and products in this chapter. Please note some skin care products containing high levels of active ingredients need to be prescribed or purchased from a doctor, dermatologist, laser clinic, beautician or cosmetic physician but there are some over-the-counter/online options too. I have included some skin care products that are natural or mostly natural and free of parabens, SLS and artificial fragrance, for those who prefer strictly chemical-free products, and these are denoted by (N) after the brand name. To find your nearest stockist you can refer to a brand's official website (see 'Resources', p. 235).

As some skin care products can be expensive, it can be helpful to read consumer product reviews online (see 'Resources' on p. 234 for review websites) before you buy. You also can test the products in-store or request product samples from the manufacturer, if available. If you are fussy about chemical ingredients check the list of ingredients of a particular product before you buy — these are usually listed online. Remember that everyone's skin is different and it's often a case of trial and error until you find the perfect match for you, but keep looking as the right skin care products can really make a difference to your skin.

What to look for

There are literally thousands of skin care ingredients so what do you look for when buying a product? When your skin is young, you might just pop a bit of shea butter moisturiser on your skin and you're set for the day. However, as you age you find the basic products might moisturise your skin but they don't reduce real signs of ageing — namely wrinkles, sun spots, mottled pigmentation, and creases on your chest when you wake in the morning! Thankfully scientists from around the globe who have an interest in skin care have determined the most *active* ingredients in skin care today.

Here are the top 5 *active* skin care ingredients for creating younger skin.

1. Retinol

Retinol is a pure form of vitamin A that improves the texture and appearance of ageing skin. Clinical trials consistently show that topically applied retinol stimulates the production of new collagen in the skin and glycosaminoglycans (GAGs), which hold water and have a plumping effect on the skin.[1] Retinyl palmitate is one of the main antioxidants found naturally in the skin and it helps to guard against the damaging effects of free radicals and UV radiation. However, this natural antioxidant depletes every time your skin is exposed to sunlight, so it's vital to restore vitamin A levels within the skin each day, especially as you age. When shopping for face moisturisers or treatments look for names such as *retinol*, *retinyl palmitate*, *retinoic acid*, *adapalene* and *tretinoin* in the list of ingredients.

Benefits of retinol in skin care*	Guidelines
stimulates production of procollagen and collagen	improvement within 28 days; best results in 24 weeks to 12 months (if using low dose and working up to a stronger dose)
increases glycosaminoglycans (GAGs)	
increases dermal matrix of skin	suitable for most skin types but sensitive skin may need time to adjust or begin on a low dose; do not apply over eczema, skin rashes or broken skin
minimises fine lines and wrinkles	
repairs some sun-induced skin ageing	
improves functioning of skin cells	wear a hat and/or use sunscreen daily when using retinol products
firmer skin (when added to cellulite products)	
decreases skin roughness	
increases protection from ulcer formation	

*Topical 0.4% retinol lotion was applied on the skin of elderly patients three times a week for 24 weeks to obtain results.[2]

High-dose retinol can irritate the skin so it's advisable to start on a low dose and acclimatise your skin, especially if you have sensitive skin. Some research shows that lower doses are just as effective as the higher prescription-only doses. Brands include Synergie (N) 'Ultimate A' serum (plus 'Reclaim' or 'Hydrolock' to moisturise), One Skin System (N) 'Vital Night Regenerate' and 'Daily Hydrate', La Mav Organic Skin Science (N) 'Bio VA5 Daily Wrinkle Smoothing Crème' and Arcona (N) 'Vitamin A Complex'. Products that offer a gradual increase of retinol include the AVST range (1 to 5) by Environ. (Refer to online product review websites listed in 'Resources' on p. 234.)

2. AHAs and BHA

As you age, your skin-cell turnover rate decreases by 30 to 50 per cent, which causes a build-up of dead skin cells. Alpha hydroxy acids (AHAs) and salicylic acid (BHA) speed up skin-cell renewal by helping to remove the substances that hold dead skin cells together and they have an exfoliating effect so your skin is left feeling smoother and softer. AHAs and BHA in skin care also improve the skin's texture by forcing the skin to renew itself more quickly than it normally would *without* damaging the skin's protective barrier. They work by setting off a *wound-healing response* in the dermis layer of the skin, which triggers increased collagen production. The eventual result is a visible reduction in sun-damaged skin, fewer wrinkles and a more even skin tone.

AHAs and BHA can help to reduce acne scars but it won't happen overnight and long-term use is necessary. Salicylic acid (BHA) is an excellent ingredient within pimple cream formulas as it reduces swelling and speeds up healing but don't apply too much as salicylic acid can temporarily dry out the skin.

Benefits of AHAs and BHA	Guidelines
skin exfoliation*	improvement within 28 days but best results with long-term use; can use an AHA peel product once a week for maintenance
increases epidermal thickness^	
improves elastic fibres (longer, thicker, less fragmented)^	suitable for most skin types (dry to oily skin), use with caution as peeling and redness can occur and don't apply to eczema or very sensitive skin
increases cell proliferation#	
increases collagen production#	don't use BHA if you are allergic to aspirin or salicylates
softer and smoother skin texture	
reduces fine lines and wrinkles	glycolic acid may increase wrinkles if overused (limit to once a week); lactic acid and malic acid are gentler with hydrating properties – ideal for dry and ageing skin
treats dry and rough skin	
reduces blemishes and acne[3]	
reduces blackheads	
reduces pigmentation and discolouration	

*Treatment with 4% glycolic acid applied twice daily for 3 weeks to healthy humans.[4]

^Treatment with 15% glycolic acid for 6 months on the facial skin of postmenopausal women.[5]

#Cultured human skin fibroblasts were treated for 24 hours with glycolic acid and malic acid. The range of cell proliferation and collagen production was significantly higher with glycolic acid treatment than with malic acid or placebo.[6]

AHAs may be listed as *glycolic acid*, *lactic acid* or *malic acid* and research shows 5 to 15 per cent concentrations offer best results. For BHA in skin care, look for the ingredient *salicylic acid* — 1 to 2 per cent concentrations are effective. Products containing more than 8 per cent AHA or BHA are sold by dermatologists, laser clinics, beauticians and cosmetic physicians and can also be given in the form of chemical peels.

AHAs and BHA can cause the skin to temporarily peel, flake and look inflamed, which is to be expected, but this can often be avoided by using lactic acid or malic acid instead of glycolic acid and by applying the product sparingly. Most products sold in cosmetic department stores have only 4 per cent or less AHA/BHA.

Brands with AHAs include Synergie (N) 'Reveal Exfoliation Serum' and 'Blem-X', One Skin System (N) 'Renewal Cleanse' (cleanser), Arcona (N) 'Vitamin A Complex'. Products with BHA include Synergie (N) 'Reveal Exfoliation Serum', and John Plunkett's 'Superfade Cream' and 'Superfade Accelerator' (for age spots and pigmentation). (Refer to online product review websites listed in 'Resources' on p. 234.)

3. Resveratrol

Resveratrol, a unique antioxidant present in the skin of red grapes, red wine, blueberries, mulberries and cranberries, has an impressive range of anti-ageing properties. Dietary resveratrol significantly inhibits AGE formation and lab studies show it has the ability to block chemically induced skin cancers from forming.[7,8]

The role of resveratrol in skin care products has been of great interest to researchers as resveratrol-based skin care formulations show 17 times greater antioxidant activity than ones containing idebenone — a popular ingredient which is closely related to coenzyme Q10.[9] As it has shown signs of blocking skin cancers from forming, the research on resveratrol has sparked the interest of skin care manufacturers who are now using the ingredient in moisturisers and sunscreens, in addition to standard UV blockers such as zinc oxide.

Benefits of resveratrol	Guidelines
potent antioxidant effect[10]	best results with long-term use.
reduces oxidative stress	suitable for all skin types (very dry to oily skin)
inhibits AGE formation[11]	
may reduce risk of skin cancers[12]	
anti-inflammatory	
antibacterial, anti-fungal and anti-viral	
useful addition to sunscreen products	

Products containing resveratrol include Environ's 'AVST' (1 to 5) range, 100 Percent Pure (N) 'Luminous Primer Vitamins + Antioxidants with Resveratrol' (note: a primer is not a moisturiser, it's for improving make-up application), Arcona (N) 'Vitamin A Complex' and 'Booster Defense Serum', and Replenix 'Ultra Sheer Sunscreen SPF 55'. (Refer to online product review websites listed in 'Resources' on p. 234.)

4. Vitamin C

A potent antioxidant in the skin, vitamin C (ascorbic acid) promotes collagen production and enhances the skin repair process. UV sunlight depletes the level of vitamin C in the skin and topical products containing antioxidants can help to replenish the skin and boost daily protection against UV rays.

Benefits of vitamin C	Guidelines
promotes collagen production[13]	use daily in the morning, best results with long-term use
reduces wrinkle formation[14]	
boosts effectiveness of vitamin E[15]	may cause irritation in sensitive skin; do not apply over rosacea, acne, eczema or rashes
speeds wound healing and repair	
stimulates dermal fibroblasts for synthesis of collagen	ascorbic acid is unstable in water-based products so products usually have a short shelf life; pure L-ascorbic acid crystals that you mix with moisturiser before application ensures potency
reduces UV/sun damage[16]	
reduces skin pigmentation over long term	

Vitamin C in skin care products may be listed as ascorbic acid, L-ascorbate or ascorbyl palmitate. Brands include Synergie (N) 'Suprema-C Serum' or 'Pure C 100%' mixed with a serum/cream that suits your skin type), One Skin System (N) 'Vital Night Regenerate' and 'Ultimate Vitamin Treatment', La Mav Organic Skin Science (N) 'Bio-A7 Firming Eye Lotion' and 'Daily Vitamin-C Brightening Serum', Beauty Without Cruelty (N) 'Vitamin C Vitality Serum (with CoQ10)', and 100 Percent Pure (N) 'Nourishing Facial Oil'. (Refer to online product review websites listed in 'Resources' on p. 234.)

5. Zinc oxide and other sunscreen filters

UV sun damage is the biggest threat to younger skin so it's essential to have skin care that offers protection from the sun's rays. One of the best sunscreen filters is zinc oxide as it guards against UVB and UVA sun damage. Topical products containing zinc oxide can also accelerate wound healing and repair skin cells, and zinc creams lock in moisture during the wound healing process (and it's a common ingredient in calamine lotion and nappy rash creams). Zinc oxide can have a drying effect on the skin so it is most suitable for normal to oily skin types.

Benefits of zinc oxide	Guidelines
treats skin rashes reflects UV rays protects against sun damage reduces risk of premature wrinkles long-term use can reduce skin pigmentation assists wound healing	apply sunscreen daily to face, hands, neck and chest/décolletage; use mineral make-up or moisturisers with SPF30+ or higher (SPF15 is not high enough) look for sunscreen that is labelled 'broad spectrum' suitable for most skin types; if you have very dry skin, zinc oxide may make your skin feel drier

Brands include Eco Logical Skin Care (N) 'Eco Face SPF30+ Sunscreen' and 'Eco Body SPF30+ Sunscreen'.

For dry skin types: Synergie (N) 'Uberzinc Essential Daily Moisturiser', and Skinstitut 'Age Defence SPF50+' which can be used on the face, hands, neck and chest.

For those who cannot use liquid sunscreens due to breakouts there are sunscreens in mineral powder form such as Synergie Minerals 'Second Skin Crush' (make-up with SPF), Colorescience Pro 'Sunforgettable Mineral Powder' SPF30 or SPF50 or Peter Thomas Roth 'Instant Mineral SPF30'. (Refer to online product review websites listed in 'Resources' on p. 234.)

A note on vitamin D

Vitamin D is manufactured in the skin after direct sunlight exposure and it's also obtained through your diet. It's a fat-soluble vitamin that directly and indirectly controls more than 200 genes so it's important your skin makes enough of it. Sunscreens block the production of vitamin D and while your face, hands, neck and chest should be protected with sunscreen at all times when outdoors, give your body some early morning sun exposure before applying sunscreen. About 10 minutes of direct sunlight in the morning or later in the afternoon, when the sun is not at its hottest and most damaging, is enough to boost vitamin D production in the skin.

Also eat vitamin D-rich foods such as fish and other seafoods. Vitamin D deficiency symptoms are listed on p. 93.

Other useful skin care ingredients

The following is a list of ingredients that are useful in general skin care products such as cleansers, hand creams, body lotions, liquid hand soaps and body washes.

Apple cider vinegar. ACV is an effective disinfectant, helps to restore the acidic pH to the skin and treats dandruff (add a splash to your shampoo along with a dash of tea tree oil to make a dandruff remedy). Add a teaspoon of ACV to a bowl of water and use as a facial wash to restore pH, or add 2 tablespoons to bathwater for a pH balancing bath. Note that ACV is acidic so make sure you dilute it before use.

Blackcurrant seed oil. Rich in gamma linolenic acid (GLA) and omega-3, it's anti-inflammatory and has moisturising properties. Suitable for dry, irritated and sensitive skin conditions (not oily or acne-prone). Products include REN 'Hydra-Calm Global Protection Day Cream' and 'Hydra-Calm Cleansing Milk'. (Refer to online product review website listed in 'Resources' on p. 234.)

Calendula. An anti-inflammatory and calming ingredient, it stimulates the production of collagen. Products include Synergie (N) 'Reclaim', Jurlique (N) 'Calendula Cream' (for irritated skin), Avalon Organics (N) 'Hand and Body Lotion' and 'Lemon Bath and Shower Gel'.

Evening primrose oil. Contains gamma linolenic acid (GLA) which is anti-inflammatory. Suitable for dry skin conditions and inflamed skin prone to eczema. Products include Synergie (N) 'Uberzinc' face moisturiser, sunscreen and primer.

Green tea. Contains polyphenols which can suppress some forms of UV-induced skin cancers. Brands include La Mav Organic Skin Science (N) 'Hydra Calm Cleansing Crème' (cleanser), Synergie (N) 'Uberzinc' and Kosmea (N) 'Eighth Natural Wonder Revitalising Facial Serum'.

Lecithin. A natural emulsifier and humectant with moisturising properties, it attracts moisture to the skin and is a natural part of skin cell membranes. Used in many skin care products such as Jurlique (N) 'Jasmine Body Care Lotion'.

Vitamin E (d-alpha tocopherol). A potent antioxidant to protect skin against free radicals, vitamin E also protects skin care products from free-radical formation. Vitamin E is in most moisturiser products, such as Sukin (N) 'Cream Cleanser' and Dr.Organic 'Pomegranate Body Butter'. Avoid synthetic vitamin E which is identifiable by 'dl' (dl-alpha tocopherol).

Caution: *100 per cent* vitamin E oil can cause hyperpigmentation (unattractive browning of the skin) if you use it over scars or directly on the skin. *This does not occur in skin care with added vitamin E — problems only occur with the pure oil.* Don't use a combination of vitamin E and selenium as there is increased risk of hyperpigmentation (also avoid oral supplements of combined selenium and vitamin E). 100 per cent vitamin E oil nearly made the next list because of its potential to cause hyperpigmentation.

Top skin care ingredients to avoid

There are many skin care ingredients that you can avoid if you prefer natural or organic products, however this list contains the top two — chosen above all others because they can enhance the ageing effect.

Sodium lauryl sulfate (SLS)

Sodium lauryl sulfate is the most widely researched skin care irritant and it's often used to purposely damage the skin's protective barrier function in experiments. SLS damage can be seen under a microscope for up to 4 weeks after use and 9 days by the naked eye. Products containing SLS create poor skin barrier function, causing excess water loss from the skin, making it easier for other chemicals, dust mites and bacteria to penetrate the skin. SLS can cause reactions such as rashes, dandruff, hair loss and dry skin (and rebound oily skin and enlarged pores).

SLS is found in many foaming toiletries such as commercial toothpastes, shampoos, cleansers, handwash and bubble bath — in most products that bubble and foam. Similar problematic ingredients are listed as:

- sodium C14-16 olefin sulfate
- sodium laureth sulfate — often in baby products!
- TEA-lauryl sulfate.

Look for products that are 'sulfate-free' or 'SLS-free' — there are many at health food shops and they are becoming increasingly popular in supermarkets and other retail outlets. Brands that have SLS-free wash products include Avalon Organics and Sukin.

Petroleum jelly

Petroleum jelly (petrolatum) was first discovered in the 1800s in some of America's first oil rigs; however, today's petroleum jelly is more refined and a vastly improved product. It is often recommended to combat painful, dry skin conditions and to seal in moisture for skin conditions such as eczema or psoriasis (it is fine to use sparingly on the body for these conditions).

However, this ingredient poses a number of problems for the skin *on your face*. Facial use of petroleum jelly can make you look older — it enlarges pores around your nose, causes rebound excessive dryness after you stop using it, and it visibly *increases the growth of facial hair*. You do not want excessive facial hair if you are a woman. Once you have increased facial hair growth it may not be reversible (should I repeat this?) but if this occurs speak to a beautician for advice, as waxing or laser are options.

Avoid using these products as face moisturisers: Vaseline, pawpaw ointment (the petroleum varieties) and avoid any skin care products that have a Vaseline-like consistency (check ingredients and online reviews).

FAQ: 'I'm on a budget and I can't afford to buy lots of skin care products. What do you suggest?'

If you can only add a couple of super anti-ageing products into your routine I'd suggest a daily face moisturiser with added retinol as it's a good long-term investment for your skin and a treatment containing high-dose AHAs to encourage cell turnover and collagen production. And use any type of sunscreen that is 20+ or higher (sun protection is most important so anything is better than nothing).

A cheap body moisturiser, as long as it's antioxidant-rich, such as Avalon Organics 'Hand and Body Lotion' range will help guard against oxidative damage, ageing and sun damage. Also, if you are in Australia or New Zealand buy Australian or locally made products as they are cheaper than the imported brands.

FAQ: 'I have very dry and sensitive skin. Vitamin A and AHAs cause irritation. What should I use?'

Products containing retinol, glycolic acid or salicylic acid may initially cause irritation so avoid them if you have sensitive skin. If you have a reaction, remove the product and apply a heavy-duty dry skin moisturiser over the top, such as Weleda (N) 'Skin Food' (this is super thick and greasy and can also be useful for dry hands and chapped skin). Also look for skin care products which are specially formulated for dry and sensitive skin, check skin care reviews online and if possible test products before purchase.

Skin care regime

Now that we've discussed the best and worst ingredients to look out for in skin care products, let's look at your morning and evening skin care regimes.

Morning face care ritual

1. Rinse face and neck with water.*

2. Optional: if you have blemishes, sparingly apply a BHA/salicylic acid product to the affected areas; or if you have hyperpigmentation apply a lightening product or AHA product to the affected area/s.

3. Apply face moisturiser with added vitamin C

4. Put on sunscreen or mineral make-up with SPF 20 or higher.

*In the morning, only cleanse with a gentle skin cleanser if necessary as you don't want to wash away your skin's protective oils too often.

Applying moisturiser and anti-ageing products

Pat the moisturiser onto your skin rather than rubbing — you will use less product, which can save you money and reduce wastage. Patting is also a more gentle way to handle the skin and this pressing motion helps to relax your facial muscles, which may reduce stress-related wrinkles.

Morning body care routine

- ✸ Apply body moisturiser (one with added antioxidants) after showering; products include Avalon Organics (N) 'Hand and Body Lotion', Synergie (N) 'B-juvenate', Dr.Organic 'Pomegranate Body Butter', Yes to Blueberries 'Rejuvenating Body Lotion' and Yes to Carrots 'Super Rich Body Butter'.
- ✸ Apply sunscreen to hands, neck and chest if not covered by clothing.
- ✸ Other parts of the body need 10 minutes of direct sunlight exposure to produce vitamin D in the skin, then afterwards, if you are spending long periods in the sun, apply sunscreen to the rest of your body.

Evening face care ritual

1. Cleanse skin and remove make-up (a good cleanser should not make the skin feel tight or dry — if it does, the product is too harsh).
2. Apply moisturiser with added retinol (begin with low-dose retinol with added antioxidants) or use every second night if you have sensitive skin.

Additional face care: once a week, use an AHA product to exfoliate the skin Refer to the AHA section on p. 100.

Evening body care routine

- ✸ Shower if desired.
- ✸ If you have aged hands, neck or chest apply a serum, moisturiser or treatment containing retinol, vitamin C or AHAs. Alternatively, apply a general body moisturiser that contains antioxidants.

Additional body care:

- ✸ Once a week, do Foot Soak + Scrub or exfoliate the feet with a pumice stone in the shower (see p. 113).
- ✸ Once a week, exfoliate your body using an exfoliating mitt and a gentle body wash (see opposite).

Tip: your skin care routine should suit your lifestyle, your skin type and your budget.

Exfoliating your skin

There are several types of exfoliators for the skin: AHA products, exfoliation mitts, dry skin brushing (using a specially designed long-handled brush so you can reach your back) and exfoliating scrubs (in the form of creams or gels) that contain granules or beads. These microscopic beads 'polish' the skin as you rub them in a circular motion and are most commonly used in face exfoliating products.

Exfoliating removes dead skin cells that tend to look flaky and dry so your skin will appear more smooth and hydrated after exfoliating. Your skin may be a little red afterwards, especially if you have sensitive skin — so be gentle. The best time to exfoliate is at night, before bed, as any skin redness will subside during sleep.

It's not absolutely essential to exfoliate but if you have dry skin, flaky skin, blackheads, wrinkles and premature ageing or if you need to remove the last remnants of fake tan, then a granulated cream or a quick scrub will leave your body or face looking and feeling softer and visibly smoother. However, you must take care not to use harsh exfoliators that can scratch the delicate skin on your face.

Alpha hydroxy acid (AHA) products not only exfoliate the skin, with long-term use they also trigger collagen renewal and can reduce enlarged pores and blackheads. AHA products may not be suitable if you have sensitive skin. Always remember to use sunscreen products during the day if AHAs are a part of your skin care routine.

If you have sensitive skin and would like to use a facial exfoliator, choose one with spherical beads (such as the jojoba exfoliator made by REN Clean Skincare) as they're gentler than ones made from apricot kernels. For the body you can use mitts, natural body scrubs or dry skin brushing. Don't forget to exfoliate your knees, knuckles, elbows and feet.

Tip: don't exfoliate your skin if you have acne as it may spread pimples, and avoid going over broken skin such as wounds, bites or rashes such as eczema.

How to use a body exfoliator

Have a quick shower. Then spread a generous amount of scrub onto your damp skin — or use an exfoliating mitt with a gentle non-SLS body wash — and massage with circular motions. Start at the feet and work your way up towards the heart (this is also how you use the exfoliator mitts). Then exfoliate from your hands to your shoulders, your chest and as much of your back as possible (a dry-skin brush is useful for exfoliating the back). Rinse thoroughly with water (by showering) and then moisturise. Your body should feel deliciously soft!

An inexpensive way to exfoliate your body (but not your face) is to use exfoliating mitts or by dry-skin brushing with a long-handled body brush. If you're using an exfoliator mitt or glove (which feels rough like Velcro), wet the mitt first, then apply a natural body wash or gel to the mitt, then exfoliate your damp skin and rinse off the body wash.

Body wash

The skin has a protective acid mantle so it's best to use gentle body washes, handwash and cleansers that are *pH balanced* or that contain acidic ingredients such as *lemon* or *apple cider vinegar*. Labelling will state if the product is pH balanced or look for gentle liquid soaps that are SLS or *sulfate-free*.

Products include Avalon Organics 'Lemon Bath and Shower Gel' (N). Health food shops usually have suitable products; just ask for assistance if you need advice.

Tip: add a tiny amount of apple cider vinegar to your hand- and body-wash products at home — less than a teaspoon will do.

Foot Soak + Scrub

DO THIS WEEKLY FOR BEAUTIFUL FEET!

Feet are often neglected and they can develop all types of unattractive problems later in life such as cracked heels and hard calluses. To remove dead skin, minimise calluses and have younger, more beautiful feet do this routine at least once a week. If you don't have time, buy a pumice stone from the pharmacy and use it weekly to exfoliate your feet in the shower — it's so important to scrub your feet and pumice stones are the best. Read the notes before you begin. You will need:

warm water

1 or 2 tablespoons apple cider vinegar

1 pumice stone (one that is new and not shared with other family members)

foot/hand or body moisturiser

Place warm water into a large, wide bowl and add vinegar. Place the bowl onto a towel on the floor where you can comfortably sit and soak your feet for 5 minutes. Then use a pumice stone, rubbing it on the soles of your feet in a circular motion. Concentrate on the hard, callused areas but don't overdo it the first time. Wash your feet and dry them, then apply moisturiser (you might need to wipe off excess before walking or avoid moisturising the bottom of your feet if there is a risk of slipping).

NOTES

❉ If you have tinea or any infection on your feet or nails, treat the condition before you use a pumice stone as you may contaminate the pumice stone and you will need to buy a new one if this occurs. Try using tea tree oil or something prescribed by your doctor or pharmacist and wait until symptoms disappear before using the foot scrub recipe.

Make-up for younger skin

The use of cosmetics dates back to 1200 BC, when the Ancient Egyptians — who had versions of most of today's make-up products — used it to enhance facial attractiveness.[17] Researchers at Harvard University found that women feel more confident when wearing make-up; it increases people's perceptions of a woman's warmth, competence and trustworthiness, and it makes a woman appear younger — provided the make-up is not trashy or poorly applied. [18]

There are exceptions to every rule, however, and some women look more attractive without make-up, and some don't like using cosmetics and that is fine too. If you like using make-up, here are some tips for a younger, more flawless finish.

Primer

Applied after moisturiser, a liquid primer fills crevices and helps concealer and foundation to glide on seamlessly for a flawless finish and a more youthful appearance. The only downside is that some primers can cause next-day breakouts if you are prone to them — if this occurs, discontinue use and avoid silicon-containing primers.

How to use: wash your hands (to remove any bacteria from them) then apply primer to one area at a time. While it's still wet, apply concealer on your problem spots and blend it in. Avoid putting too much around your eyes as your make-up may move. Primers can cause next-day break-outs and they are often filled with artificial chemicals, but an alternative is to use your regular moisturiser as a primer, just before applying your make-up. Brands include 100% Pure (N) 'Luminous Primer Vitamins + Antioxidants with Resveratrol'. Check online product reviews for more information.

Concealer

A concealer product can be used to hide dark circles under the eyes, blemishes and hyperpigmentation. Use sparingly after primer, avoid using over wrinkles and favour products that are lightweight (such as Yves Saint Laurent 'Radiant Touch'). If you have red patches, use a green corrector concealer (CoverGirl

makes a cheap one), blend then cover with a sheer powder mineral make-up —
remember, less is more.

Foundation

Foundation makes you look younger *if it's not too obvious*. It improves facial
symmetry and evens out skin texture and tone.

How to use: sparingly, as a concealer or very lightly as you do not want to
look as if you are wearing a mask. Poorly applied foundation can accentuate your
wrinkles so apply less, avoid foundations that have either too much shimmer or
are too matte, and if applying liquid foundation, use a flat, square make-up brush
that doesn't soak up (and waste) your make-up, such as MAC 191, or a cheaper
equivalent. Apply to your face and partway down your neck, if the colour is
perfectly matched to your skin, and blend well. Reduce the shine with blotting
paper or a tissue, or sparingly use powder applied with a quality mineral make-
up brush.

Eye make-up

Unless you are a pro at applying eye shadow, keep your eye make-up simple. You
will need two basics: an eyelash curler to 'open up' the eyes and a super lash-
extending mascara — only in black — such as Maybelline 'Illegal Length'. Replace
your mascara frequently — every 2 months — as bacteria can build up over time.

Bronzer

Powdered or liquid bronzers are used to darken the face and neck, and to even
out the skin tone. However, bronzing products can make people look older
(much older!) and they can go on patchy if you have dry, rough or wrinkled
skin. If you are over the age of 30, it's often best to avoid bronzers or, if necessary,
apply them sparingly to give your skin a hint of 'natural' colour (as opposed to
an artificial tanned look).

Quality bronzing powder is best used to even out the skin tone: for example,
use it on your neck if it needs darkening to match the tone of your face or if
you have patchy skin that needs evening out. Remember, less is best. Also avoid

using fake tan on your face as it can dry out the skin and accentuate wrinkles. If you are fair skinned, *your face should be slightly lighter than your body* to give the appearance of younger skin.

Tips

Before buying a make-up product, apply some from a tester and then *go outside* and look at your skin in natural light to check if the product matches your skin tone and looks natural. Always do your make-up in good or natural light and re-check your make-up once you are outdoors (such as when you are in your car) to see if it has been applied correctly.

Lipstick

French researchers found that wearing lipstick can make women appear healthier. However, avoid brown or dull-coloured lipsticks, avoid shimmer tones and high gloss (unless you are under 25) and enlist the advice of an expert about colour choice for your skin type. How you apply the lipstick is very important as a bumpy lip line can make you look a little dishevelled.

How to use: lipstick often goes on smoother if you first apply a small amount of liquid foundation to your lips, then blend it out towards the skin around your mouth until it is almost invisible and then blot with a tissue. This will reduce the risk of the lipstick bleeding into any nearby wrinkles, and it gives you a blank canvas to work with. Ensure the lip line is perfect by using a lipstick brush to apply the lipstick (this is the best choice) or alternatively use a matching pencil to outline. If your lipstick starts caking later in the day, wipe it off, repeat the foundation step (which will help lipstick more effectively 'stick' to your lips) and reapply.

Beautifully applied make-up — that looks natural and highlights your features — can hide age spots and whatever else your diet and skin care regime cannot fix. I highly recommend investing in a make-up book and having a make-up lesson from an expert. Free make-up consultations are often available from speciality make-up stores such as MAC, Mecca Cosmetica and Napoleon Perdis (or in the cosmetics section of larger department stores). Look for make-up books written specifically for your age group (see Rae Morris in 'Resources', p. 233).

Face steaming, to relax the face

The face holds tension and muscle contractions can, over time, contribute to wrinkles. It can help to consciously relax your face daily, and steaming your face before bed can help (and it can help promote a more restful night's sleep). You will need:

1 large bowl (or use the basin, provided it is clean)
very warm water
small splash of apple cider vinegar
1 large clean cotton cloth/face washer

After cleansing your face and rinsing off the cleanser, fill a bowl with very warm water. Add a small amount of apple cider vinegar — the vinegar is an optional step that is designed to help restore the acid mantle of the skin. Wet your cloth and quickly wring out the excess water. Then hold the cloth against your face and gently press, imagining your facial muscles relaxing each time you breathe out. Hold the cloth over your face for 5–10 seconds and repeat the process three times.

Part 2

The 28-day program

Chapter 8

How this program works

The 28-day program for younger skin works by incorporating each of the following factors into your daily routine. Each one helps the other to work more effectively.

Diagram 4: How the Younger Skin program works

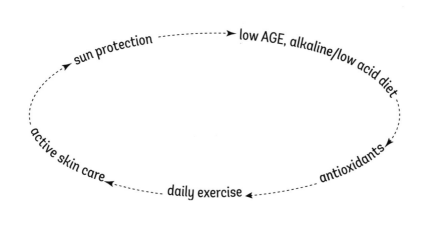

Here are the top 5 steps for younger skin in more detail.

1. Low AGE, alkaline/low acid diet

When combined, a low AGE diet and a low acid (or increased alkaline) diet offers you the best chance at creating younger skin. The average Western diet is rich in acid-promoting foods and AGEs and both cause premature ageing of the skin.

A quick look at AGEs in your diet

❊ Foods that are *very low* in AGEs include wholegrains, rice, tea and herbal teas, raw vegetables and most fruits.

❊ *Low to medium* dietary AGEs include grilled vegetables, coconut milk, raw fish (sushi), vegie burgers, chicken or fish which has been marinated, poached or steamed with a little lemon added to the water.

❊ *High* dietary AGEs are found in skinless chicken and most cooked fish — the recipes in this book will show you how to reduce the AGE content of these foods.

❊ *Very high* dietary AGEs are found in butter, margarine, cheeses, red meat, chicken skin, sausages, deli meats and bacon. These are the main foods you should avoid during the 28-day program.

A list of foods containing AGEs in varying amounts can be found on pp. 222–223.

A quick look at acidifying and alkalising foods

❊ *Highly alkalising* foods are wonderful for the skin and these include lemon, lime, beetroot, apple cider vinegar, sprouts and dark leafy greens.

❊ *Alkalising* foods are good for the skin and these include avocado, raw almonds, banana and most vegetables.

❊ *Acidifying foods* include wholegrains, most fruits, most seafoods, tofu, chicken, legumes and cooked tomato — these are fine to eat in moderation.

❄ *Highly acidifying* foods include beef, pork, processed junk food, sugar, white bread, deli meats, margarine, soft drink/sodas and alcohol — these should be avoided during the 28-day program.

A complete list of alkalising and acidifying foods can be found on pp. 226–231.

The menus and recipes in this book show you how to shop for and prepare foods that are lower in AGEs and are acid–alkaline balanced. The recipes also show how you can protect meats with marinades and by cooking with liquids and lower temperatures.

The diet works together with the next four factors to create younger skin.

2. Antioxidants

Antioxidants protect against oxidation of skin cells and they reduce AGE formation in the body. You can obtain antioxidant protection through both supplementation and foods such as fruits, vegetables and seeds — especially the ones that are red, purple or black. The most important antioxidants such as vitamin C, zinc and anthocyanins should ideally be obtained from your diet (additional supplementation might be required if you have deficiency signs — the Nutrient Deficiency Questionnaire on p. 90 can help you identify possible deficiencies).

3. Exercise

Frequent exercise has a protective effect against AGE formation and it speeds up wound healing in older adults.[1,2] Exercise reduces inflammation, normalises glucose metabolism and improves blood flow to the surface of your skin, giving your skin a natural, healthy glow. Daily exercise, enough to cause you to sweat, flushes microbes from the surface of your skin and assists with the removal of waste products from your body. It's also one of the keys to minimising the appearance of cellulite.

Exercise daily for 28 days — frequent, medium-impact movement is a vital part of this program and it will give you glowing, healthy skin. See FAQs on p. 131 for the best forms of exercise to try.

4. Skin care

Skin care products that contain *active* ingredients do more than moisturise your skin — they also encourage cell renewal, increase GAGs (which offer support and hydration), increase the dermal matrix of skin and minimise fine lines and wrinkles. Some active ingredients improve the skin's texture by forcing the skin to renew itself more quickly than it normally would. They work by setting off a *wound-healing response* in the dermis layer of the skin, which triggers increased collagen production. Your diet works hand-in-hand to supply all the nutrients needed for this collagen renewing process. Turn to the previous chapter for more details.

5. Sun protection

Frequent UV exposure is the number one cause of wrinkles. Sun exposure causes the formation of AGEs in the skin, which paralyse collagen fibres and reduce skin elasticity.[3] The sun depletes vitamin A in the skin, damages GAGs (which offer support and hydration) and triggers the appearance of MMPs, which degrade collagen and elastic fibres.

No matter how perfect your diet or how many antioxidants you consume, it will be for naught if you don't use sun protection on the main ageing zones: your face, neck, hands and chest. During the next 28 days, *wear a hat and use sunscreen* — they are the best anti-ageing weapons (if you don't like liquid sunscreen there are non-liquid options too, covered on p. 105). Hat information starts on p. 35.

8 tips for younger skin (you might not have thought of)

Here are eight more tips you might want to employ to help you look your best.

Sleep on your back

Researchers from Turkey studied people with oblique or horizontal wrinkles on their face and found they all had one thing in common: they slept in a prone position with their face buried into their pillow.[4] If you find sleeping on your back difficult, *cuddle a pillow over your heart* as it promotes a secure feeling that enables your body to relax.

Don't oversleep

For beauty sleep, have 7 to 8 hours of quality sleep each night but don't sleep for longer. Oversleeping promotes dehydrated skin and a study found that more than 8 hours of sleep each night can shorten your lifespan.[5]

Steam your face before bed

Frown lines between the eyebrows and crow's feet at the corners of the eyes are thought to be caused by small muscle contractions. Your face can be incredibly tense without you realising it and habitual facial expressions such as squinting and frowning eventually leave their mark. 'Face steaming' helps to relax facial muscles and promotes better sleep, and it's described on p. 117.

Dress beautifully and be well groomed

British researchers demonstrated how ill-fitting or plain clothing can age a 55-year-old woman by seven years. In contrast, they found *a well-cut wardrobe* (quality fabrics, stylish and well-fitting garments) sheds up to eight years from a woman's face — that's a total of fifteen years younger!

Wear driving gloves

While driving, your hands are exposed to direct sunlight for long periods and gloves serve to protect your hands from sun exposure, age spots and wrinkled fingers. American researchers found that sunlight coming in through the driver's side of the car can contribute to skin cancer development on that particular side of your body.[6] A total of 92 per cent of skin cancers occur on the sun-exposed areas of the head, neck, arms and hands so protect these while driving.[7]

Don't worry so much

Stress causes the release of the stress chemical adrenaline, which inhibits proper digestion, and cortisol increases blood sugar levels and promotes collagen loss. The result is prematurely aged skin and 'frown lines' between your eyebrows.

Laugh and smile more

The faces of happy people look three years younger than non-smiling people, according to German researchers.[8]

Wear make-up, but keep it classy

A study published in the *Journal of Applied Social Psychology* revealed that women who wear cosmetics are perceived as being healthier and more youthful than when they are bare faced.[9] Researchers from Harvard University found that wearing make-up not only boosts a woman's attractiveness, it also increases people's perceptions of her likability, her competence and trustworthiness — provided the make-up looks classy and is applied correctly. (See 'Make-up for younger skin' in Chapter 7).

Chapter 9

Frequently asked questions

Read this chapter before you begin the 28-day program to find answers to the most commonly asked questions, from the amount of food you should be eating, to food choices when dining out and the type of exercise that's best for your skin.

FAQ: 'How much should I eat?'

Eat three main meals and a couple of snacks each day. Avoid skipping meals as this can mess with your blood sugar levels and promote fatigue and sugar cravings (and sugar bingeing, which is bad for your skin). Here are some guidelines:

Breakfast: Your serving size can vary but it's important to eat something healthy that fills you up so you have enough energy to get you through until lunch. The menus, beginning on p. 144, will give you some healthy choices.

Lunch and dinner: Fill half your plate with vegetables, one quarter with quality protein such as chicken, fish or legumes and the other quarter with quality carbohydrates such as sweet potato, basmati rice, quinoa or spelt — see the diagram below. If you want to avoid carbohydrates at night you can consume extra vegetables in place of grains with your dinner.

Diagram 5: How much food should go on your plate?

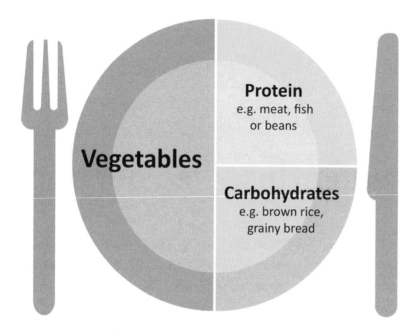

Dessert: Favour antioxidant-rich fruits such as guava, banana, papaya, pawpaw or berries of any kind (frozen mixed berries are great) or try the smoothie recipes, which start on p. 164.

Don't go hungry. There are plenty of delicious recipes and foods to choose from so stock the fridge with healthy ingredients before you begin the 28-day program. The menus, which begin on p. 144, and the shopping list, on p. 214, will show you what to do.

FAQ: 'Do I need to strictly follow the 14-day menu?'

This is a flexible program so if you have allergies or aversions you can adapt the menus to suit. You can also adjust the program to suit your skin by referring to the Skin

Problem Chart, which starts on p. 216. If you prefer not to follow the menus, you can refer to the recipes, in Chapter 11, and design a program to suit your tastes.

FAQ: 'How much coffee and tea can I drink?'

Ideally, you should avoid drinking coffee or strong black tea as they are highly acid-producing and rich in caffeine. However, this is a flexible program which allows one or two cups of coffee or black tea daily as they are low in AGEs and a morning cuppa can be an essential ritual for some people. Favour herbal teas (there are recipes starting on p. 166) or chai tea (the leaf variety, not the powder) as it has some caffeine but also contains alkalising ginger, cinnamon and cloves so has a balance of acid and alkaline ingredients. If you drink a coffee or tea I suggest either exercise afterwards, drink a vegetable juice or eat a salad to restore the acid–alkaline balance to your diet.

FAQ: 'What can I eat when I'm out at restaurants and cafes?'

Sushi and Thai food are good choices. Thai cooking, where vegetables are stir-fried briefly, should only contain low to medium AGEs and other vegetarian options are usually lowest in AGEs (along as they are cheese-free). Avoid deep-fried foods, beef and pork. Avoid curries that have been cooking for hours (vegetarian may be okay). Other options include:

- salads
- soups (no dairy/cream/cheese)
- casseroles, tagines, stews
- raw sushi
- vegetable curries (no dairy/cream)
- Thai stir-fried vegetables
- fish with steamed vegetables
- rice (not fried rice)
- seafood marinara (tomato based, no cream)
- dahl or other lentil dishes (no cream or cheese).

FAQ: 'I'm always craving sugar, bread and alcohol, what should I do?'

All three of these products supply the body with glucose for energy but they are not in a desirable form that will give you a steady supply and you will soon crave more (an unhealthy cycle that is bad for your skin!). Sugar cravings can indicate the following:

- ❋ Your body may be low in vitamin C, which is packaged in sweet fruits (hence the biological craving for something sweet).
- ❋ If you have just eaten a high salt meal, your body's electrolytes may be out of balance and your body is craving potassium — from fruit. The correct salt and potassium levels in your body are essential for normal function of your cells and organs — so if you happen to eat a salty meal, grab a potassium-rich banana, peach or papaya for dessert.
- ❋ It can indicate blood sugar problems requiring chromium or cinnamon in the diet (which must be taken at the same time as eating carbohydrates to be most effective).
- ❋ Other factors such as lack of sleep, overworking or skipping meals can cause sugar cravings.

Cravings for bread and other carbohydrates can indicate the need for a chromium and magnesium supplement to help with blood sugar control. Cravings for alcohol can indicate the need for magnesium (and counselling, if necessary). If you have an insatiable craving for sugar or carbohydrates, eat quality low GI grains such as Omega Muesli (p. 169) or grab a piece of antioxidant-rich fruit — two to three pieces daily is recommended. Fruit is a guilt-free way to have a sweet treat and get your daily dose of AGE-reducing super-nutrients at the same time. The best fruits for younger skin are listed in the handy shopping guide on p. 214.

FAQ: 'Will I have to avoid pan-frying or baking foods during the 28 days?'

For centuries frying and baking have been popular cooking methods so you do not need to avoid these. The recipe section will show you how to fry and bake foods in a slightly different way that minimises AGE formation during cooking.

FAQ: 'What types of exercise are best for the skin?'

You have two aims when exercising: to sweat and to tone your muscles so your skin pulls back to the muscle and appears to be firmer. Walking on a flat surface is not effective at toning and building muscle, and unless it's uphill and on a hot day you will not sweat enough either. So unless you are injured or frail and cannot do much exercise, it's best to try some medium-impact exercise that incorporates toning your problem areas (which are commonly the arms, stomach, thighs and bottom).

Below is a list of some of the best forms of exercise for younger skin.

* Soft sand jogging/walking is ideal because the surface is unstable so it calls upon the stabilising muscles, which are the smaller muscles that control balance, promote core strength and act to keep certain parts of the body steady so that the primary working muscles can do their job properly — the result is increased toning of the skin (and the softer surface is kinder to your joints than jogging on hard surfaces).

* Boxing and using weights are great for toning the arms (just be careful not to jar your neck while throwing punches).

* After having a baby you can use a post-pregnancy workout DVD (such as The Tracy Anderson Method) to tone problem areas, or speak with a personal trainer.

* Speak with an exercise coach or a personal trainer about your problem areas and have a program designed for you. An exercise coach can show you how to get results fast and avoid injuries along the way. Check the Internet for personal trainers, exercise classes and fitness groups in your local area. It's always best to try to find a teacher or personal trainer who has professionally accredited qualifications, so look for certification from the governing body for your chosen style of exercise.

FAQ: 'I am 25 years old and I already have good skin, will I notice a difference on the program?'

If you already have young skin then you won't see dramatic results. However, the program will teach you how to care for your skin and body so it looks its best for many years to come.

FAQ: 'I have eczema and my skin is frequently irritated, so is this 28-day program right for me?'

If you have eczema, multiple food sensitivities, skin rashes or irritated skin, this program may be unsuitable for you, especially while you are experiencing flare-ups. The program detailed in my book *The Eczema Diet* would be better for you to begin with, then after your eczema has improved you can begin the 28-day program for younger skin (see 'Resources', p. 233, for more information).

FAQ: 'My new skin care routine has caused my skin to flake; what should I do?'

If your skin is flaking, dampen your skin and wet a soft wash cloth, then gently rub your skin in circular motions to remove the peeling skin (however, do not rub your skin if it's red or irritated). If you have very dry skin, apply a hydrating moisturiser a few minutes after applying active skin care products such as serums. The flaking should subside within 3 days and your skin will feel smooth and soft.

Do not apply AHAs and active skin care products onto eczema or irritated skin. It is recommended to have a professional prescribe high strength products to you, so you buy the right products for your skin type (and budget!), and they can show you how to apply the products for maximum results and minimal irritation, if any.

FAQ: 'My skin has broken out, what should I do?'

Breakouts can occur early in the program for several reasons:

1. If you are not used to eating plenty of fresh vegetables, or a cleansing diet, then you may experience typical detox symptoms. Fatigue and breakouts can occur as your body is eliminating an increased amount of toxins and these symptoms should subside within a week. Just ensure you are drinking plenty of hydrating liquids.

2. A new moisturiser or a cleanser that is too oily or not right for your skin type can cause breakouts and these will subside quickly with a change in products. Also avoid make-up primers and liquid sunscreens if you find they cause pimples (powdered sunscreens are an alternative, and you can use your daily moisturiser as make-up primer).

3. Active ingredients such as AHAs and vitamin C can cause temporary breakouts as they activate deep cleansing within the skin — this is okay and symptoms should stop within a week. However, if a product continually causes pimples, stinging, redness or rashes then discontinue use.

4. Stress can trigger breakouts, so seek advice on managing stress, worry, anxiety, etc.

5. Eating a food that is not right for your skin type can trigger breakouts in some individuals. If you are prone to acne, oily skin or minor breakouts, reduce your intake of fats. Avoid cooking oils, rice bran oil (extra virgin olive oil may be okay in moderation), flaxseed oil, linseeds/flaxseeds, LSA, nuts (especially almonds), almond milk, and red meats (saturated fat) as they increase oil content in the skin. If breakouts occur, use skin care products with added salicylic acid, formulated for treating pimples, and drink more water.

FAQ: 'Do I really need to drink lots of water?'

Yes. Drink eight glasses of hydrating liquids daily, including filtered water, herbal teas and fresh vegetable juices.

FAQ: 'What are the main foods to avoid during the 28-day program?'

The main foods and beverages to avoid during the 28-day program — and for younger skin — include dairy products, wheat, refined sugar, alcohol and red meat. If you have been diagnosed with an iron deficiency you can add *lean lamb* to your diet as prescribed by your doctor (lamb is lower in AGEs and has a lower acid-producing effect than beef).

Other foods to avoid include artificial additives, most cooking oils and margarine. I also recommend you avoid grapefruit and grapefruit juice as they block phase 1 liver detoxification and this causes increased chemicals, medical drugs (if taking) and hormones to stay in the blood, which can lead to skin problems (and health complications if taking medications or drugs or if drinking alcohol).

Avoid any foods and drinks that cause adverse reactions — these include allergy foods, food sensitivities and foods that cause you to bloat (or cause any other unpleasant symptom). It is not a gluten-free program but if you are allergic to gluten there are simple adjustments you can make to the program. The 28-day program is designed to meet all the nutritional needs of a healthy adult so if you have a wide range of foods to which you are allergic, if you are ill or are a fussy eater, it's best to speak with a nutritionist or other health care professional about your diet.

FAQ: 'During the first week will I experience a detox effect?'

The 3-day Alkalising Cleanse is designed to greatly improve detoxification of chemicals so temporary symptoms such as increased tiredness and changes in the skin may occur. If you have an overgrowth of candida albicans, either on the skin or in the mouth or digestive tract, you might experience irritability and tiredness, as well as increased cravings for sugar. This should pass quickly. Just ensure you drink plenty of water and if you want to reduce any detox symptoms you can reduce your intake of the Anti-ageing Broth and vegetable juices.

FAQ: 'What if I have a negative reaction to a food?'

You could have a unique allergy so take note if a food makes you feel unwell or itchy. In this case you may need to vary the menu so you are eating different foods each week or introduce one new food every 3 days, if you are not used to new products such as linseeds/flaxseeds or pomegranate. If you have introduced a range of new products at once (e.g. if you are using a new skin cream plus consuming flaxseed oil and spelt bread) and you experience symptoms, suspect an allergy or an intolerance and go back to the 'one new food/product every 3 days' rule — that is, only introduce one new food or product every 3 days, thus giving you time to see if you will have an adverse reaction before introducing another new food or product. This will help you to find what's right for you.

FAQ: 'I may have gluten intolerance. Is the diet suitable for me?'

The 28-day program is a wheat-free diet but it's not gluten-free. If you are sensitive to gluten you will need to avoid wheat, oats, rye, barley, spelt, regular soy milk and other products containing gluten. Substitute with rice, buckwheat, chickpeas or beans, linseeds/flaxseeds, lentils, quinoa, malt-free soy milk (or almond milk) and gluten-free pasta. If you suspect you are gluten intolerant speak with your doctor about testing for coeliac disease.

FAQ: 'I'm vegetarian so can I follow the 28-day diet?'

If you are vegetarian or vegan you can follow the program, just use vegetarian protein substitutes such as legumes, beans, almonds, tofu and tempeh, with grains such as basmati rice and red quinoa to make your meals more complete in protein. Avoid vegetarian products such as vegan sausages that contain artificial flavour enhancers and preservatives. Also avoid drinking tea with your meals as the tannins bind with iron and can slowly cause iron deficiency, especially if you don't eat meat.

Ensure you don't have an iron or vitamin B12 deficiency *before you begin* the program (see p. 90 for the questionnaire or have your doctor do a blood test). During the program eat plenty of iron-containing green leafy vegetables, oat cereals with added iron, beans, lentils, wholemeal pasta, tofu and wholemeal spelt bread, along with vitamin C-rich fruits such as guava, papaya and lemon to enhance iron absorption — the 14-day menu starting on p. 140 will help you do this.

FAQ: 'I'm quite thin and I don't want to lose weight; do I need to modify the program?'

The 28-day menu can cause weight loss if you are not used to eating cleansing or healthy foods. Thin people may need to eat an extra meal each day to maintain their weight, such as Omega Muesli for dessert (p. 169). Ensure you are having quality carbohydrates with each meal (rice, oats, barley, sweet potato, spelt pasta), smoothies for snacks or add avocado to lunches.

FAQ: 'What should I do after the 28-day program to keep my skin looking good?'

To ensure your skin stays beautiful, you can continue with several basic principles from the program. The most important ones are:

1. Eat *purple foods* on most days, such as blueberries and other berries, eggplant (aubergine), purple carrots and red cabbage or add a side of mixed purple and green salad leaves to your lunch or dinner, as they are rich in chlorophyll for healthy skin. If you have a garden, plant some red lettuce, blueberries and purple basil (whatever is most suitable for your climate or area) so you have a supply of anthocyanin-rich foods on hand.

2. Eat vitamin C-rich *red and orange* foods daily, including guava, sweet potato, papaya, pawpaw, peach, capsicum (pepper) or carrots.

3. Use *low-AGE cooking methods* such as steaming or poaching with added lemon. Cook meats in marinades, soups and stews or at reduced temperatures, and add alkalising lemon and lime to your drinks and meals. Drink herbal teas, filtered water and fresh vegetable juices often.

4. *Exercise* three to six times a week — it is essential for toning the skin.

5. Continue using 'active' *skin care products* and gradually increase the strength of your retinol-containing products over time (it may take up to a year for your skin to tolerate high strength retinol). Wear sunscreen and a hat to protect your face, neck, chest and hands from future sun damage — sun care is essential for beautiful skin beyond age 40.

6. For firmer, younger skin, continue to take a calcium supplement with magnesium, vitamin D, zinc and manganese (and copper, if necessary). And for blood sugar balance take a chromium supplement or simply add a sprinkle of cinnamon when eating grains and other carbohydrates.

As the 28-day program is a balanced and healthy food-based program it can also be followed for the long term, if desired, and if you want to incorporate some extra meals into your routine, a list of health food books containing suitable recipes can be found in the Resources section on p. 233.

Chapter 10

14-day menu

This is a sample menu designed for adults with ageing skin. It begins with a 3-day Alkalising Cleanse, where you eat foods with predominantly alkalising ingredients to enhance liver detoxification of chemicals and to cleanse the digestive tract — it's low AGE too and really great for the skin. This food-based cleanse is a part of a 14-day meal plan which is repeated to make it a 28-day program (so you do the cleanse twice). If you are frail, unwell, pregnant, breastfeeding or suffering from a medical condition requiring medications you should skip the 3-day Alkalising Cleanse as it is a detox program.

The following table lists the recipes that are included in Chapter 11, as well as some general snack options for you. Next to each recipe you'll find a guide to which skin types the recipe is most suitable for. Note that when it says 'normal to very dry skin' this means the recipe contains ingredients that boost the sebum and moisture content of the skin and it may not be suitable for people with oily or blemish-prone skin.

Recipe list and snack options

Marinades	Suitable for which skin types?
Tamari, Lycopene and Lemon Marinade, p. 151 (chicken or tofu)	all skin types
Coconut and Lime Marinade, p. 152 (fish, chicken or tofu	all skin types
Tamari, Lime and Ginger Marinade, p. 152 (fish, chicken or tofu)	all skin types
Anchovy and Mustard Marinade, p. 151 (fish or chicken)	normal to very dry skin
Peach, Thyme and Chilli Marinade, p. 150 (fish, chicken or tofu)	all skin types

Dressings, dips and spreads	Suitable for which skin types?
Halo Dressing, p. 154	normal to very dry skin
Anchovy and Mustard Dressing, p. 155	all skin types
Beetroot and Almond Dip, p. 156	normal to very dry skin
Avocado and Thyme Dip, p. 155	all skin types
Almond Pesto, p. 157	dry to very dry skin
Hummus Dip, p. 153	all skin types
Ginger and Lime Dipping Sauce, p. 157	all skin types
Banana Carob Spread, p. 158	all skin types

Snack options	Suitable for which skin types?
Vegetable Platter, p. 160	best snack for all skin types
Papaya Cups with Lime and Guava, p. 159	all skin types
Lime and Berry Iceblocks, p. 159	all skin types
handful of *raw* almonds	normal to very dry skin
and 2 Brazil nuts (for selenium)	
½ dozen oysters, once a week (for zinc, copper)	all skin types
2–3 pieces of fruit daily:	all skin types (esp. acne)
choose from guava, Kumatoes,	all skin types
¼ cup blueberries or raspberries,	(avoid fruits that cause bloating)
1 cup of cherries or red seedless grapes,	
banana (not sugar variety), green apple,	
red apple (not pink lady), apricot,	
pomegranate (it's best in salads),	
peach and ½ mango.	

Drink options	Suitable for which skin types?
Cucumber and Mint Juice, p. 161	all skin types
Green Glow Juice, p. 162	all skin types
Purple Carrot Juice, p. 163	all skin types
Moisture Boost Smoothie, p. 164	dry to very dry skin
Flaxseed Lemon Drink, p. 165	normal to very dry skin
Banana, Lemon and Coconut Smoothie, p. 162	normal to very dry skin
Green Water, p. 164	all skin types
Dandelion Tea, p. 166	all skin types
Lemon and Ginger Tea, p. 166	all skin types
Lemon and Mint Tea, p. 167	all skin types
Chai Tea with Clove, p. 167	all skin types
Almond Milk, p. 168	dry to very dry skin

Breakfast options	Suitable for which skin types?
Omega Muesli, p. 169	all skin types
Berry Porridge, p. 170	all skin types
Quinoa Porridge, p. 171	normal to very dry skin
Perfect Poached Eggs, p. 172	all skin types
Boiled Eggs, p. 173	all skin types
Scrambled Eggs with Watercress, p. 174	all skin types

Lunch and dinner options	Suitable for which skin types?
Anti-ageing Broth, p. 176	all skin types
Shiitake Vegetable Soup, p. 178	all skin types
Spiced Sweet Potato Soup, p. 175	all skin types
Chicken and Barley Soup, p. 180	all skin types
Watercress Soup, p. 182	all skin types
Mediterranean Seafood Soup, p. 206	all skin types
Parcel Baked Fish, p. 184	all skin types
Sushi Rolls with Black Sesame, p. 186	all skin types
Beetroot and Carrot Salad, p. 181	all skin types
Guava and Rocket Salad, p. 188	all skin types
Winter Spiced Dahl, p. 190	all skin types
Spelt Flat Bread, p. 192	all skin types
Lemon Thyme Pizza, p. 194	normal to very dry skin
Chicken and Zucchini Pizza, p. 195	all skin types
Mixed Salad Wrap, p. 197	all skin types
Eggplant and Cauliflower Curry, p. 189	all skin types
Moroccan Lemon Chicken, p. 198	all skin types
Sweet Potato Salad, p. 200	all skin types
Shiitake Vegetable Casserole, p. 202	all skin types
Quinoa and Pomegranate Salad, p. 203	all skin types
Mango and Black Sesame Salad, p. 205	all skin types
Oregano Chicken Sticks, p. 208	normal to very dry skin
Steamed Chicken and Mint Meatballs, p. 210	all skin types
Steamed Fish with Lime and Ginger, p. 212	all skin types

On the following pages is a suggested eating plan for the 28-day program, starting with the 3-day Alkalising Cleanse. If you plan to eat the soups or dahl during the 3-day cleanse, pre-make Anti-ageing Broth (p. 176) *the day before* you start day 1. Also pre-soak your quinoa the night before, for making Quinoa Porridge on day 1, and use red quinoa, instead of white. It is recommended to pre-soak the quinoa each day; if you forget you can still make Quinoa Porridge without soaking, it will just take a bit longer.

Alkalising drinks

For 28 days *consume three alkalising drinks daily*. There will be some suggestions in the menus but after a few days you can choose your favourite drinks. Alkalising drinks include: Flaxseed Lemon Drink (p. 165); Cucumber and Mint Juice (p. 161); Green Glow Juice (p. 162); Purple Carrot Juice (p. 163); and herbal teas such as Dandelion Tea (p. 166); Lemon and Ginger Tea (p. 166); Lemon and Mint Tea (p. 167); peppermint tea and chamomile tea (no caffeine during the 3-day cleanse: no coffee, green tea, white tea or black tea, including chai). Refer to the recipe list earlier in this chapter to check which drinks are most suitable for your skin type.

Days 1 to 3

The first 3 days of the 28-day program consist of the 3-day Alkalising Cleanse. During this time drink plenty of filtered water and eat raw vegetables daily: carrot and celery sticks, sprouts, broccoli, mixed leaf salads.

Don't go hungry — eat as much soup and as many raw vegies as you like. It's also important to rest and to not go out socialising during the cleanse as you need to avoid all other foods for 3 days, and have 7 to 8 hours of quality sleep at night.

Snacks during the cleanse include Vegetable Platter (p. 160); Papaya Cups with Lime and Guava (p. 159); a handful of *raw* almonds and 2 to 4 Brazil nuts daily.

If taking supplements, have your calcium and chromium supplements twice a day with breakfast and lunch or according to the manufacturer or as prescribed. If you are a woman you need to consume about 18mg of iron daily so I recommend you take a natural, herbal iron supplement. An iron supplement is also essential if you are vegetarian or vegan (see 'Resources' on p. 233 and food sources of iron on p. 87).

Days 1 to 3: the 3-day Alkalising Cleanse

Breakfast	Lunch	Dinner
Exercise for 30–60 mins Pre-soak the quinoa: Quinoa Porridge, p. 171 Have 2–3 of the following: Lemon and Ginger Tea*, p. 166; Flaxseed Lemon Drink, p. 165; Green Water*, p. 164; Green Glow Juice, p. 162; or Purple Carrot Juice, p. 163 (no caffeine for 3 days)	Choose from: Sweet Potato Salad, p. 200; Shiitake Vegetable Soup*, p. 178; Spiced Sweet Potato Soup, p. 175; or Watercress Soup, p. 182 Drink 6 cups filtered water daily	Choose from: Sweet Potato Salad, p. 200; Shiitake Vegetable Soup*, p. 178; Spiced Sweet Potato Soup, p. 175; Watercress Soup, p. 182; or Winter Spiced Dahl, p. 190 Vitamin C-rich fruits: Papaya Cups with Lime and Guava*, p. 159 (1 serve daily) *On day 3, soak the oats if using for day 4's breakfast*

*For busy people: the fastest or easiest recipes are denoted with an asterisk in the menus.

Day 4

Breakfast	Lunch	Dinner
Exercise for 40–60 mins Choose from: Omega Muesli*, p. 169 (pre-soak oats); or Scrambled Eggs with Watercress, p. 174 Tea of choice, and Green Water*, p. 164; or Cucumber and Mint Juice, p. 161 (have 2–3 alkalising drinks daily, listed on p. 226)	Choose from: Quinoa and Pomegranate Salad, p. 203; or Mixed Salad Wrap, p. 197; or use up leftovers* Drink 4–6 cups filtered water daily	Choose from: Parcel Baked Fish, p. 184; or Eggplant and Cauliflower Curry*, p. 189; or use up leftovers Vitamin C-rich dessert: Papaya Cups with Lime and Guava*, p. 159

Day 5

Breakfast	Lunch	Dinner
Exercise for 40–60 mins Choose from: Berry Porridge, p. 170; or Quinoa Porridge, p. 171 Tea of choice; Green Water*, p. 164; or Green Glow Juice, p. 162 (2–3 alkalising drinks daily)	Choose from: Quinoa and Pomegranate Salad, p. 203; or Mixed Salad Wrap, p. 197; or use up leftovers* Afternoon snack: Vegetable Platter, p. 160; or fruit (berries or cherries) Drink 4–6 cups filtered water daily	Choose from: Moroccan Lemon Chicken, p. 198; or Shiitake Vegetable Casserole*, p. 202; or use up leftovers* *Soak the oats for tomorrow's breakfast; pre-freeze 2 bananas (peel them first) for smoothies*

Day 6

Breakfast	Lunch	Dinner
Exercise for 40–60 mins Choose from: Omega Muesli*, p. 169; or Quinoa Porridge, p. 171 Tea of choice*; Purple Carrot Juice, p. 163 (2–3 alkalising drinks daily)	Choose from: Sweet Potato Salad, p. 200; or Mixed Salad Wrap, p. 197; or soup of choice* Afternoon snack: Vegetable Platter, p. 160; or fruit (guava, papaya or peach) Drink 4–6 cups filtered water daily	Choose from: Winter Spiced Dahl, p. 190; or use up leftovers* Optional dessert: Moisture Boost Smoothie, p. 164; or a banana *Make a double batch of Lime and Berry Iceblocks, p. 159, for next week*

Day 7: treat day

Breakfast	Lunch	Dinner
Exercise for 40–60 mins Choose from: Scrambled Eggs with Watercress*, p. 174; or Banana, Lemon and Coconut Smoothie, p. 162 Chai Tea with Clove*, p. 167 and 2–3 alkalising drinks (list on p. 226)	Choose from: sushi* (store-bought); Sushi Rolls with Black Sesame, p. 186; or use up leftovers* Afternoon snack: Vegetable Platter, p. 160; or fruit (berries or cherries) Drink 4–6 cups filtered water daily	Choose from: Mediterranean Seafood Soup, p. 206; or Lemon Thyme Pizza with a side of mixed salad leaves, p. 194; or restaurant option* (listed on p. 129) Lime and Berry Iceblock; or Papaya Cups with Lime and Guava, p. 159

Day 8

Breakfast	Lunch	Dinner
Exercise for 40–60 mins Choose from: Omega Muesli*, p. 169; or Quinoa Porridge, p. 171 Tea of choice*; Cucumber and Mint Juice, p. 161 (2–3 alkalising drinks daily)	Choose from: Quinoa and Pomegranate Salad, p. 203; or Mixed Salad Wrap, p. 197; or use up leftovers* Drink 4–6 cups filtered water daily	Choose from: Steamed Chicken and Mint Meatballs, p. 210, with steamed greens or salad; or soup of choice* Lime and Berry Iceblock; or fruit (banana or peach)

Day 9

Breakfast	Lunch	Dinner
Exercise for 40–60 mins	Choose from: Beetroot and Carrot Salad with Spelt Flat Bread, p. 181; or sushi* (store-bought); or Mango and Black Sesame Salad, p. 186	Choose from: Shiitake Vegetable Soup*, p. 178; or Eggplant and Cauliflower Curry*, p. 189
Choose from: Perfect Poached Eggs with spelt bread, p. 172; Boiled Eggs, p. 173; or Omega Muesli*, p. 169	Drink 4–6 cups filtered water daily	Lime and Berry Iceblock*, p. 159
Tea of choice; Green Water*, p. 164; Green Glow Juice, p. 162 (2–3 alkalising drinks daily)		*Soak the oats or quinoa for tomorrow's breakfast; pre-freeze 2 bananas (peel them first)*

Day 10

Breakfast	Lunch	Dinner
Exercise for 40–60 mins	Choose from: Mixed Salad Wrap, p. 197; or Quinoa and Pomegranate Salad, p. 203	Choose from: Steamed Fish with Lime and Ginger, p. 212; or Spiced Sweet Potato Soup, p. 175
Choose from: Omega Muesli*, p. 169; Quinoa Porridge, p. 171; or Moisture Boost Smoothie, p. 164	Drink 4–6 cups filtered water daily	Vitamin C-rich dessert: Papaya Cups with Lime and Guava*, p. 159
Tea of choice*; Purple Carrot Juice, p. 163 (2–3 alkalising drinks daily)		

Day 11

Breakfast	Lunch	Dinner
Exercise for 40–60 mins	Choose from: Mixed Salad Wrap, p. 197; or Quinoa and Pomegranate Salad, p. 203	Choose from: Oregano Chicken Sticks, p. 208; or Watercress Soup, p. 182
Choose from: Omega Muesli*, p. 169; or Quinoa Porridge, p. 171	Drink 4–6 cups filtered water daily	Lime and Berry Iceblock*, p. 159; or Moisture Boost Smoothie, p. 164
Tea of choice*; Purple Carrot Juice, p. 163 (2–3 alkalising drinks daily)		

Day 12

Breakfast	Lunch	Dinner
Exercise for 40-60 mins Choose from: Perfect Poached Eggs with spelt bread, p. 172; Boiled Eggs, p. 173; or Omega Muesli*, p. 169 Tea of choice; Green Water*, p. 164; Green Glow Juice, p. 162 (2-3 alkalising drinks daily)	Choose from: Sweet Potato Salad, p. 200; or Mixed Salad Wrap, p. 197; or use up leftovers* Afternoon snack: Vegetable Platter, p. 160 Drink 4-6 cups filtered water daily	Choose from: Mediterranean Seafood Soup; p. 206; soup of choice; or leftovers* Fruit: papaya and cherries or sliced apple *Soak the oats and peel and freeze 2 bananas for tomorrow, if using*

Day 13

Breakfast	Lunch	Dinner
Exercise for 40-60 mins Choose from: Omega Muesli*, p. 169; or Moisture Boost Smoothie, p. 164 Tea of choice*; Cucumber and Mint Juice, p. 161 (2-3 alkalising drinks daily)	Choose from: Guava and Rocket Salad, p. 188; Mixed Salad Wrap, p. 197; or soup of choice* (Shiitake Vegetable Soup*, p. 178, leave out mushrooms if desired) Drink 4-6 cups filtered water daily	Choose from: Chicken and Barley Soup*, p. 180; or leftovers* Fruit: papaya and cherries or sliced apple or Moisture Boost Smoothie, p. 164

Day 14

Breakfast	Lunch	Dinner
Exercise for 40-60 mins Choose from: Scrambled Eggs with Watercress*, p. 174; or Banana, Lemon and Coconut Smoothie, p. 162 Tea of choice* and 2-3 alkalising drinks daily	Choose from: Sweet Potato Salad, p. 200; Mixed Salad Wrap, p, 197; or soup of choice* Afternoon snack: Vegetable Platter, p. 160; fruit (berries or cherries) Drink 4-6 cups filtered water daily	Choose from: Shiitake Vegetable Casserole, p. 202 (without shiitake mushrooms if desired); or Lemon Thyme Pizza, p. 194, with Mango and Black Sesame Salad, p. 205 Lime and Berry Iceblock*, p. 159; or Moisture Boost Smoothie , p. 164

Day 15 onwards: repeat the 14-day menu, also read FAQs in Chapter 9 if you haven't already.

Conversion table

Oven temperatures

°Celsius (C)	°Fahrenheit (F)
120	250
150	300
180	355
200	400
220	450

Cup and spoon conversions

1 teaspoon	5ml
1 tablespoon	20ml
¼ cup	60ml
⅓ cup	80ml
½ cup	125ml
⅔ cup	160ml
¾ cup	180ml
1 cup	250ml

Volume equivalents

Metric	Imperial (approximate)
20ml	½fl oz
60ml	2fl oz
80ml	3fl oz
125ml	4½fl oz
160ml	5½fl oz
180ml	6fl oz
250ml	9fl oz
375ml	13fl oz
500ml	18fl oz
750ml	1½ pints
1L	1¾ pints

Weight equivalents

Metric	Imperial (approximate)
10g	⅓oz
50g	2oz
80g	3oz
100g	3½oz
150g	5oz
175g	6oz
250g	9oz
375g	13oz
500g	1lb
750g	1⅔lb
1kg	2lb

Abbreviations

V+Vn	vegetarian and vegan option
GF	gluten-free
HF	ingredient usually available in health food sections of larger grocery stores or from health food shops

Chapter 11

Recipes

Unusual ingredients + substitutes

Ingredient	What is it and where do I buy it?	Substitute product
apple cider vinegar	the only vinegar which is alkalising; organic is best (preferably not double strength); HF	apple cider vinegar: halve the dosage if using double strength
black sesame seeds	anthocyanin-rich sesame seeds; they're not toasted but taste like it; HF	white sesame seeds but they don't offer the same benefits
rice malt syrup	natural sweetener (the only one that is alkalising); HF	yellow box honey (it's low GI) or agave nectar
tahini (hulled tahini paste)	paste made with sesame seeds, hulled varieties taste best; HF	If making hummus, you can make it tahini-free by using more water, lemon juice and oil. If spreading onto bread, substitute with mashed avocado.
tamari	wheat-free and gluten-free soy sauce; favour reduced salt varieties with no flavour enhancers; HF	soy sauce (contains wheat), favour reduced salt with no added MSG or flavour enhancers

Marinades

Flavoursome marinades that contain a combination of acidic ingredients such as lemon and lime protect protein foods from excessive AGE formation during cooking. Marinades are also wonderful for adding flavour to foods such as seafood, fish, meats and tofu. Please note that the following marinades are best used immediately before cooking and you do not need to leave the meats to marinade for hours beforehand.

Peach, Thyme and Chilli Marinade

MAKES ¾ CUP; PREPARATION TIME 5 MINUTES

This delicate and faintly sweet marinade is rich in antioxidants and complements chicken and fish. Save a couple of tablespoons to use as a decorative sauce for fish or a dipping sauce for prawns.

½ lemon, juiced (you need 40 ml/1⅓fl oz)

2 ripe peaches, seeds removed and chopped

1 tablespoon fresh oregano leaves, finely chopped

1 tablespoon fresh lemon thyme leaves

sprinkle of quality sea salt and ground black pepper

½ small red chilli or sprinkle of chilli flakes

Using a food processor or blender, blend the lemon, peach, oregano, lemon thyme and a sprinkle of salt and pepper. Taste and add a little chilli at a time until the desired heat is achieved. Pour over chicken or fish, mix and cook immediately, if desired. For tender chicken or fish, cook in parcels (Parcel Baked Fish recipe, on p. 184, can be adapted for chicken).

NOTES

✸ Variations: add 1 tablespoon freshly grated ginger or use nectarine instead of peach.

Anchovy and Mustard Marinade

MAKES 1 SERVE; PREPARATION TIME 5 MINUTES

Ideal for marinating fish and chicken.

6 anchovy fillets, drained

¼ cup milk (soy milk or other)

2 tablespoons rice bran oil

1 tablespoon wholegrain mustard

½ lemon, juiced (approx. 1 tablespoon juice)

Place the anchovies in milk to reduce the fish flavour. After about a minute, remove the fish from the milk, and rinse the anchovies. Discard the milk.

Blend the anchovies, oil, mustard and lemon in a small food processor until combined. Alternatively, finely slice the anchovies and mash with a fork, then combine with the other ingredients and mix well.

Tamari, Lycopene and Lemon Marinade

MAKES ENOUGH FOR 2–3 MEALS; PREPARATION TIME 5 MINUTES

Tomato sauce is rich in lycopene, while lemon supplies vitamin C and reduces AGE formation during cooking. This marinade is perfect for meats such as chicken or tofu (see Oregano Chicken Sticks on p. 208).

1 tablespoon fresh lemon juice

½ cup tamari (preferably salt-reduced)

1 tablespoon rice malt syrup or honey

4 tablespoons organic tomato sauce (ketchup)

1 teaspoon freshly grated ginger

1 teaspoon minced garlic

Mix ingredients together and pour over meat. Mix to coat the meat, then cover and refrigerate (for up to 2 hours) or use immediately.

Coconut and Lime Marinade

MAKES 1–2 SERVES; PREPARATION TIME 5 MINUTES

This Thai-style marinade goes well with tofu or fish, in recipes such as Parcel Baked Fish (p. 184).

½ cup light coconut milk

1 teaspoon finely grated fresh ginger

1 small lime, juiced (approx. 3 teaspoons fresh lime juice)

3 teaspoons tamari (preferably salt-reduced)

½ small red chilli, or chilli flakes (optional)

Mix ingredients together and pour over fish or seafood of choice and mix. Cover and refrigerate for 5 minutes then cook according to recipe instructions.

NOTES

❁ Variations: add a sprinkle of chilli flakes and freshly minced garlic.

Tamari, Lime and Ginger Marinade

MAKES 1 SERVE; PREPARATION TIME 5 MINUTES

This Thai-style marinade is perfect for meats, fish or tofu. Use on recipes such as Oregano Chicken Sticks (p. 208) or Parcel Baked Fish (p. 184).

1 tablespoon fresh lime juice

3 tablespoons tamari (preferably salt-reduced)

1 teaspoon freshly grated ginger

Mix ingredients together and pour over meat, tofu or fish and mix. Cook immediately, if desired.

NOTES

❁ Variation: add 1 tablespoon of finely chopped coriander (cilantro).

Dressings, dips and spreads

Hummus Dip

SERVES 8; PREPARATION TIME 10 MINUTES

This is a healthy, protein-rich spread that contains calcium and magnesium, and a range of antioxidants including lemon polyphenols that can help to balance blood sugar. Serve with vegetable 'dipping sticks' such as red capsicum (pepper), peeled carrot and celery, or use in place of butter on Spelt Flat Bread (p. 192).

1 x 400g (14oz) can chickpeas (or use freshly cooked: see notes)

5 tablespoons water

4 tablespoons hulled tahini

juice of ½ lemon (2–3 tablespoons juice)

2 teaspoons apple cider vinegar

1 teaspoon freshly minced garlic

1 teaspoon cumin

1 teaspoon honey (optional)

½ teaspoon paprika (sweet paprika)

quality sea salt, to season

ground black pepper, to season

Drain and rinse the chickpeas (or cook them fresh) and discard any discoloured ones, then place in a food processor. Add the remaining ingredients and blend on high speed until puréed. Add a small amount of water or extra lemon juice if the dip is too thick.

Taste the mixture and season with salt and pepper if desired. If refrigerated, hummus will stay fresh for up to a week.

NOTES

❋ If you would like to cook dried chickpeas instead of using canned chickpeas, use 200g (7oz) dried chickpeas and read 'Cooking guide for legumes' on p. 70.

Halo Dressing

MAKES 6+ SERVES; PREPARATION TIME 4 MINUTES

An alkalising salad dressing, ideal for salads and sweet potato dishes.

2 tablespoons honey (yellow box or other)

¼ cup apple cider vinegar (not double strength)

1 tablespoon flaxseed oil

2 tablespoons oil (see notes)

Place all ingredients into a jar and shake well. Taste and adjust the flavour if desired (see notes). Use 1–2 teaspoons per person on salads or baked sweet potato recipes.

NOTES

❊ If you have oily or normal skin use extra virgin olive oil, or for dry skin use rice bran oil.

❊ Flaxseed oil changes the taste of the dressing so adjust the measurements to suit your palate. Do not use flaxseed oil on hot foods as heat damages the oil.

❊ You can also add freshly minced garlic or a pinch of yellow curry powder for added antioxidants.

Anchovy and Mustard Dressing

MAKES 2 SERVES; PREPARATION TIME 5 MINUTES

This flavoursome dressing complements Sweet Potato Salad, p. 200 (or you could make a tasty niçoise salad with it).

3 anchovy fillets, drained

¼ cup milk (soy or other)

2 teaspoons extra virgin olive oil

2 teaspoons wholegrain mustard

1 tablespoon apple cider vinegar

Place the anchovies in milk to reduce the fish flavour. After about a minute, remove the fish from the milk, discard the milk and rinse the anchovies.

Blend anchovies, oil, mustard and vinegar in a small food processor until combined.

Avocado and Thyme Dip

MAKES 2 SERVES; PREPARATION TIME 4 MINUTES

This lovely alkalising dip is suitable as a spread for making sandwiches and Mixed Salad Wraps (p. 197) or for accompanying recipes such as Sweet Potato Salad (p. 200) and Vegetable Platter (p. 160).

1 ripe avocado (see avocado tips, p. 205)

2 teaspoons fresh lemon or lime juice

2 sprigs lemon thyme, leaves stripped and chopped

quality sea salt

cracked black pepper

Mash the avocado and blend in the citrus juice, then add the chopped lemon thyme leaves and season with salt and pepper.

Beetroot and Almond Dip

MAKES 1½ CUPS; PREPARATION TIME 10 MINUTES, COOKING TIME 30 MINUTES

This highly alkalising dip is rich in protein and the potent antioxidant betalain, which gives beetroots their remarkable colour. If using the leftover almond meal from making Almond Milk (p. 168), adjust the amount of water to suit — you may need less.

1 medium beetroot (approx 200g/7oz), top removed

½ cup raw almonds or ½ cup leftover almond meal

1 lemon, juiced (3 tablespoons juice)

2 tablespoons tahini paste

2–3 tablespoons filtered water

1 clove garlic, minced

½ teaspoon ground cumin

½ teaspoon quality sea salt

1 teaspoon apple cider vinegar

Wash and scrub the beetroot and place it into a small pot of boiling water. Simmer on low for 30 minutes or until soft. Meanwhile, if using raw almonds, place the almonds into a bowl of water and soak until the beetroot is ready. Drain and place the beetroot into cold water, then peel it.

Drain almonds and place them in a food processor along with the beetroot, lemon juice, tahini, water, garlic, cumin, salt and apple cider vinegar. Process until smooth, adding a little extra water if needed (a teaspoon at a time).

NOTES

❋ Variation: add 1 teaspoon of black sesame seeds for added anthocyanins and a sprinkle of cinnamon.

❋ If using whole raw almonds, you can soak them for a day or overnight to make them soft.

Almond Pesto

MAKES 1½ CUPS; PREPARATION TIME 10 MINUTES

This protein-rich, alkalising spread is perfect for special occasions. Use it as a dip for the Vegetable Platter (p. 160), spread it on spelt wraps or add it to Sweet Potato Salad (p. 200). If possible, soften the almonds by soaking them overnight or all day before preparation.

1 large bunch parsley

1 cup unsalted raw almonds

¼ cup filtered water

¼ cup extra virgin olive oil

freshly minced garlic to taste (approx. 1 teaspoon)

1 tablespoon apple cider vinegar

Celtic or quality sea salt to taste

Cut half the stems off the parsley, wash the leaves in a bowl of water and shake off excess water and place into a food processor. Add all the remaining ingredients and blend well.

NOTES

✽ Variation: if almonds give you breakouts, use raw cashews instead (cashews are not alkalising but the other ingredients are).

Ginger and Lime Dipping Sauce

MAKES 1 SERVE; PREPARATION TIME 4 MINUTES

½ lime, juiced (approx. 1 tablespoon)

1 tablespoon salt-reduced tamari

½ teaspoon freshly grated ginger (peeled first)

Combine all ingredients and serve in a small dish. Ideal with Sushi Rolls with Black Sesame (p. 186) or Steamed Chicken and Mint Meatballs (p. 210).

Banana Carob Spread

MAKES 2–3 SERVES; PREPARATION TIME 5 MINUTES

This sweet alkalising spread is rich in fibre and potassium. Use it on bread or Spelt Flat Bread (p. 192).

1 ripe medium banana, mashed

1 teaspoon carob powder

¼ avocado, mashed

Mix together the banana, carob and avocado. Spread onto quality bread or lightly toasted spelt sourdough. Store leftovers in a small jar and use within 2 days.

Snacks

Papaya Cups with Lime and Guava

SERVES 2; PREPARATION TIME 5 MINUTES

This fresh fruit cup is suitable as a light snack or healthy dessert. If available use a small red guava, or substitute with ¼ large apple guava. Do not refrigerate guava as it tastes ripe and delicious when at room temperature.

1 ripe papaya, halved and seeds removed

1 ripe guava, washed, de-seeded and sliced

½ lime, juiced

Fill the papaya halves with chopped guava and sprinkle with lime juice.

NOTES

✽ Variation: instead of guava use chopped banana. For extra antioxidants, sprinkle with black sesame seeds or flaxseeds/linseeds and add a few chopped mint leaves.

Lime and Berry Iceblocks

SERVES 6; PREPARATION TIME 5 MINUTES, ALLOW TIME TO FREEZE

Berries are rich in antioxidants and coconut water is a naturally sweet drink fresh from coconuts. With added lime juice, these iceblocks are both alkalising and rich in vitamin C for healthy skin.

½ cup frozen raspberries and/or blueberries

juice of 1 lime

2 cups coconut water (ensure it's 100% pure)

Mash the berries then divide the pureé into the base of 6 iceblock (ice lolly) moulds. Mix the lime juice and coconut water and pour over the berry pureé in the iceblock moulds and freeze overnight.

Vegetable Platter

SERVES 2; PREPARATION TIME 5 MINUTES

This platter of alkalising vegetables supplies vitamin C, carotenoids and anti-cancer indoles (an organic compound). Protein- and fibre-rich dips to choose from are: Hummus Dip (p. 153), Almond Pesto (p. 157), Beetroot and Almond Dip (p. 156) or store-bought hummus (see notes).

1 cup chopped raw broccoli (purple or green)

1 small carrot (orange or purple), peeled and sliced

½ red capsicum (pepper), sliced

dip of choice

Wash all vegetables thoroughly. Arrange on a platter and serve alongside your dip of choice.

NOTES

✸ When choosing a store-bought dip, ensure it contains no artificial preservatives (numbers), raw egg, cheese or other dairy.

✸ Variations: use celery sticks, cucumber, red cabbage or add mixed sprouts to the platter.

Drinks

Cucumber and Mint Juice

SERVES 2; PREPARATION TIME 5 MINUTES

This alkalising drink is designed to reduce inflammation, aid liver detoxification and promote a healthy skin glow.

2 medium or large cucumbers

4 celery stalks

1 knob ginger

½ bunch mint

filtered water

½ lemon, juiced

Soak the cucumbers, celery, ginger and mint in water with a splash of apple cider vinegar for 3–5 minutes then remove and drain.

Scrub the celery and ginger if needed. For a stronger ginger flavour, leave the skin on; for a milder taste, peel off the ginger skin. Trim approximately 1cm (⅓in) of the stalks from the mint.

Using a juicing machine, juice the cucumber, celery, mint and ginger, ending by adding a splash of filtered water.

Remove from machine then add the lemon juice and stir.

Green Glow Juice

SERVES 3; PREPARATION TIME 5 MINUTES

A highly alkalising juice to thin the blood and give your skin a natural glow.

½ bunch mint

5 kale leaves

5 stalks celery

2 handfuls mixed sprouts

2 green apples

apple cider vinegar

Trim approximately 1cm (¹/₃in) of the stalks from the mint. Soak the kale, celery, sprouts, apples and mint in water and a splash of apple cider vinegar for 3–5 minutes then remove and drain. Scrub celery if needed.

Using a juicing machine, juice the ingredients, ending by adding a splash of filtered water.

Banana, Lemon and Coconut Smoothie

SERVES 2; PREPARATION TIME 3 MINUTES (IF ALMOND MILK IS ALREADY MADE)

1 frozen banana, chopped (peel before freezing)

1 cup chilled coconut water

1 cup chilled Almond Milk (p. 168; or organic soy milk)

½ lemon, juiced

Place all ingredients into a blender and blend until mixture is smooth.

NOTES

❋ Variations: if your skin is oily add a few chopped mint leaves and use soy milk instead of almond milk. If your skin is dry add 1 teaspoon of flaxseed oil or chia seeds.

Purple Carrot Juice

SERVES 3; PREPARATION TIME 5 MINUTES

This sweet juice is rich in AGE-reducing anthocyanins and carotenes.

1 tablespoon apple cider vinegar

2 purple carrots (if unavailable, see notes)

2 large carrots (orange)

2 large apples (dark red if possible)

3 large stalks celery

½ cup mixed sprouts

filtered water

In a large bowl of water, place a splash of apple cider vinegar and soak the vegetables, apples and sprouts for 3–5 minutes, then remove and drain. Scrub the celery and carrots if desired.

Using a juicing machine, juice the ingredients, ending by adding a splash of filtered water.

NOTES

✺ If you cannot find purple carrots use beetroot, red cabbage or purple kale and extra carrots. Avoid raw cabbage if you have thyroid problems. Beetroot has a high GI so add cinnamon to this drink if substituting with beetroot.

Moisture Boost Smoothie

SERVES 2; PREPARATION TIME 5 MINUTES

This alkalising drink contains omega-3, anthocyanins and cryptoxanthin-rich papaya to reduce AGEs and hydrate dry, wrinkle-prone skin (it's not suitable if you have acne or oily skin conditions).

1 ripe pre-frozen banana, chopped (peel before freezing)

½ cup frozen blueberries

½ cup diced papaya

1½ cups chilled Almond Milk (p. 168; or water)

1 tablespoon fresh mint leaves, finely chopped

1 tablespoon soy lecithin granules (non-GMO)

2 teaspoons flaxseed oil or whole flaxseeds/linseeds

pinch of ground cinnamon

Place all ingredients into a blender and blend on high until smooth.

NOTES

✺ Soy lecithin granules make the oils easier to digest. Do not use lecithin if you are allergic to soy.

Green Water

SERVES 1; PREPARATION TIME 1 MINUTE

This dark green drink is highly alkalising and rich in magnesium. See notes.

1 teaspoon liquid chlorophyll

1 glass chilled filtered water (optional: chilled mineral water)

Mix together and drink.

NOTES

✺ Avoid 'double strength' or 'high concentrate' liquid chlorophyll that is blackish in colour, as this may stain the teeth with long-term use. (Grants makes a medium-strength formula that is green, not black, but other products may also be suitable — ask at your local health food shop for advice.)

Flaxseed Lemon Drink

SERVES 2–3; PREPARATION TIME 5 MINUTES

Over the years I've had great feedback about this alkalising drink, which featured in the original Healthy Skin Diet (this is a new, simple version). It's super hydrating and helps to soften the skin. If you have acne or oily skin see notes.

½ lemon, skin washed and scrubbed

2 cups chilled filtered water

2 teaspoons organic flaxseed oil

¼ teaspoon freshly grated ginger

5 mint leaves, chopped (optional)

1 tablespoon soy lecithin granules

Zest (finely grate) the skin of the lemon and place zest into a blender. Then juice the lemon and add the juice and the remaining ingredients to the blender.

Blend on high for 30 seconds or until frothy and thoroughly blended. Strain if desired. Have this drink throughout the day or before each main meal.

NOTES

✸ If you have acne or oily skin omit the flaxseed oil.

Dandelion Tea

SERVES 1; PREPARATION TIME 2 MINUTES

Dandelion root is alkalising and according to research it increases phase II liver detoxification (where your liver deactivates and removes from the body chemicals, toxins, excess hormones and pesticides) by 244 per cent. Have up to 2 cups daily to stimulate digestion. See notes.

½ teaspoon ground dandelion root

1 cup (250ml) boiled water

1 teaspoon rice malt syrup or yellow box honey

Place the dandelion root into an enclosed tea strainer. Dunk the tea strainer into boiled water and steep for about 5 seconds, until water is dark brown. Make this tea weak to begin with, as it can be quite strong in flavour. Add honey if desired.

NOTES

✸ More than 3 cups daily can overstimulate digestive acids. Dandelion tea is not suitable if you suffer from stomach ulcers or heartburn.

Lemon and Ginger Tea

SERVES 1; PREPARATION TIME 3 MINUTES, STEEPING TIME 5 MINUTES

1 cup boiling water

1 thick wedge of lemon (pre-wash and scrub lemon skin before cutting)

1 large slice fresh ginger root

1 clove

Place the freshly boiled water into a coffee mug. Squeeze the juice of the lemon into the mug and add the lemon wedge, ginger and clove. Allow to steep for 5 minutes. Optional: strain before drinking.

NOTES

✸ For sweetness add 1 teaspoon rice malt syrup or yellow box honey.

Lemon and Mint Tea

SERVES 1; PREPARATION TIME 3 MINUTES, STEEPING TIME 5 MINUTES

1 cup boiling water

1 thick wedge of lemon (pre-wash and scrub lemon skin before cutting)

3 fresh mint leaves, washed

Place the freshly boiled water into a teapot or tea cup. Squeeze the juice of the lemon into the teapot or cup and add the lemon wedge and mint leaves. Allow to steep for 5 minutes. If using a cup, remove the wedge and leaves before drinking.

Chai Tea with Clove

SERVES 1–2, PREPARATION TIME 5 MINUTES

Chai tea is a delicious antioxidant-rich tea that contains some caffeine thanks to the black tea content. Store-bought chai tea bags usually contain black tea, cinnamon, ginger, cloves and cardamom. This brew has added ginger and cloves to boost the anti-inflammatory and anti-AGEing effect. As this drink contains some caffeine, do not consume it during the 3-day cleanse.

1 cup boiling water

1 organic chai leaf tea bag

1 slice fresh ginger root (or 1 organic ginger tea bag)

1 whole clove

Place the freshly boiled water, the tea bag, ginger and clove into a teapot (or saucepan) and let it steep for 5 minutes. Strain it as you pour it into a teacup.

NOTES

❄ Variations: add organic soy milk and 1 teaspoon of rice malt syrup; or add a squeeze of fresh lemon juice or use a lemon and ginger tea bag instead of plain ginger.

Almond Milk

MAKES 6 SERVES; PREPARATION TIME 2 MINUTES + OVERNIGHT SOAKING (RECOMMENDED)

Almonds are a super food for moisturising the skin, plus they're alkalising and a source of calcium and protein for a healthy acid mantle of the skin. You can use Almond Milk instead of cow's milk in smoothies, on porridge or muesli. This recipe also has added linseeds/flaxseeds for omega-3 balance. *Almond milk is not suitable if you have oily skin, acne or eczema.*

1 cup whole raw almonds (not roasted or salted)

3 cups (750ml/1½pt) filtered water

1 tablespoon whole linseeds/flaxseeds

dash of ground cinnamon

Soak the almonds in 2 cups of water overnight (highly recommended but not essential). Drain the almonds and rinse.

Place all ingredients into a blender and blend on high for about 30 seconds. Strain the liquid, using a measuring cup to press out the last of the liquid through the strainer.

Consume the milk within 5 days.

NOTES

�֍ The leftover almond meal can be used to make Beetroot and Almond Dip (p. 156). Or use it to make a body scrub to gently exfoliate your skin.

Breakfast

Omega Muesli

SERVES 1; PREPARATION TIME 5 MINUTES + OVERNIGHT SOAKING (RECOMMENDED)

This soaked muesli dish is rich in omega-3, vitamin C, potassium and fibre. Soaking the oats and linseeds/flaxseeds overnight with apple cider vinegar (ACV) increases mineral availability and goodness, and it softens the oats so they can be eaten raw. Using ACV is optional and if you forget to soak the oats overnight just soak them for 20 minutes covered with warm water (half cool water, half boiled water from the kettle).

¾ cup rolled oats

1 teaspoon whole linseeds/flaxseeds

filtered water

sprinkle of apple cider vinegar (½ teaspoon)

chilled Almond Milk (p. 168; or organic soy milk or water)

¼ cup blueberries or berries of choice

dash of ground cinnamon

Place oats and linseeds into a bowl with enough water to cover, add a sprinkle of ACV and tightly cover with plastic wrap. Leave on the bench overnight (do not refrigerate).

The next morning, drain off the water using a strainer, rinse the oats and linseeds with filtered water and place into a serving bowl.

Add almond milk and top with berries and cinnamon.

Berry Porridge

SERVES 1; PREPARATION TIME 5 MINUTES, COOKING TIME 15 MINUTES (OVERNIGHT SOAKING IS OPTIONAL)

½ cup rolled oats

filtered water

sprinkle of apple cider vinegar (optional)

chilled Almond Milk (p. 168; or organic soy milk)

½–1 teaspoon whole linseeds/flaxseeds (optional)

¼ cup fresh blueberries (or frozen raspberries, thawed)

sprinkle of ground cinnamon

If soaking overnight, place the oats in a bowl with enough water to cover them, add a sprinkle of ACV and tightly cover with plastic wrap. Leave on the bench overnight.

The next morning, drain off the water using a strainer, rinse the oats with filtered water to remove the ACV and place them into a small saucepan. Add 1½ cups filtered water (or 1 part oats to 3 parts water) and bring to the boil. Simmer on low for 10–15 minutes, stirring occasionally, adding extra water if necessary.

Pour the cooked oats into a serving bowl and top with almond milk, linseeds, fruit and cinnamon.

Quinoa Porridge

SERVES 1; PREPARATION TIME 5 MINUTES, COOKING TIME 25 MINUTES (OVERNIGHT SOAKING OPTIONAL)

Quinoa is a nutritious gluten-free seed which cooks like a grain. Soaking the quinoa overnight is recommended to make the minerals more available, but soaking is not essential. Red quinoa contains beneficial anthocyanins and has a lower GI than white quinoa.

½ cup red or white quinoa, rinsed (do not use puffed quinoa)

filtered water, plus extra for boiling

½ teaspoon real vanilla essence or ½ vanilla bean (optional)

½ cup chilled Almond Milk (p. 168; or organic soy milk)

1 teaspoon whole linseeds/flaxseeds (optional)

fruit: blueberries, papaya, banana, cherries or raspberries

sprinkle of ground cinnamon

If soaking overnight, place the quinoa and enough water to cover in a bowl, tightly cover with plastic wrap and leave on the bench overnight.

The next morning, drain off the water using a strainer, rinse the quinoa with filtered water and place it into a saucepan. Add 1½ cups of filtered water (or 3 parts water to 1 part quinoa) and bring to the boil. Then cook over low heat until the porridge is thick and grains are tender, about 15 minutes for white quinoa and 20 minutes for red quinoa. Add the vanilla essence and milk and cook for another 5 minutes on low heat. Stir occasionally to prevent burning and add a touch more milk if necessary (you want the liquid to puff up the quinoa so it's very soft).

Pour the quinoa into a serving bowl and top with linseeds, fruit and cinnamon.

Perfect Poached Eggs

SERVES 1–2; PREPARATION TIME 4 MINUTES, COOKING TIME 5–7 MINUTES

This recipe is a healthy way to cook eggs as there is no frying involved. Eggs are a rich source of B group vitamins and protein. There is an art to cooking perfect poached eggs and these tips will turn you into a pro in no time. Serve with spelt sourdough toast and avocado if desired.

2 free range or organic eggs (approx 55g/2oz each)

1 tablespoon apple cider vinegar

Fill a small saucepan with enough water to cover the eggs. Bring to the boil and add the apple cider vinegar (the vinegar keeps the egg whites together while cooking). Turn the heat off so the bubbling stops and carefully crack the eggs into the water.

Cook with the heat off for approximately 5½ minutes for runny centred eggs or 7 minutes for hard boiled (times may vary according to size of the eggs and hotplate temperature, but after making them a couple of times you will know what cooking time works for you). Carefully and swiftly remove the eggs with a spatula/slotted spoon. If desired, rinse the vinegar from the eggs using slow-running hot water from the tap (must be only a drizzle or it will damage the eggs). Thoroughly drain the water off the eggs and serve.

Boiled Eggs

SERVES 1–2; PREPARATION TIME 5 MINUTES, COOKING TIME 5–8 MINUTES

How do you know if an egg is cooked the way you like it? Lift the egg out of the water with a spoon and if the egg shell dries immediately the egg is hard boiled; if it dries slowly then the egg yolk should be runny.

1 tablespoon white vinegar

pinch of salt

2 free range or organic eggs

Fill a small saucepan with enough water to cover eggs. Bring to the boil then add vinegar and salt (vinegar and salt prevent the shells from cracking).

Gently spoon the eggs into the water. Reduce heat to a simmer. For runny egg yolks, boil for 3 minutes (for a 59g/2oz egg), turning eggs occasionally to promote even cooking. For hard-boiled eggs, cook for 8 minutes (times will slightly vary according to the size of the egg and temperature of the hotplate).

Using a dessertspoon, carefully remove the eggs from the water. Place eggs briefly into cold water to halt the cooking and then peel shells if desired. If serving soft-boiled eggs, you can place them into egg cups and cut off the top third using a knife.

NOTES

✳ Serving suggestion: for soft-boiled eggs, sprinkle with chopped parsley and serve with toast 'dipping sticks' made with spelt bread; add Kumatoes on the side.

Scrambled Eggs with Watercress

SERVES 1; PREPARATION TIME 4 MINUTES, COOKING TIME 4 MINUTES

Scrambled eggs are a low-AGE way to serve eggs. Use quality organic or free range eggs and choose omega-3 rich ones if available. For acid–alkaline balance, serve the eggs with wilted watercress as it is highly alkalising and a good source of chlorophyll and calcium. Serve with Spelt Flat Bread (p. 192) or quality spelt sourdough bread if desired.

1 cup watercress, washed and stems trimmed

2 eggs, lightly beaten

splash of filtered water (1–2 teaspoons)

quality sea salt (optional)

You can serve the watercress uncooked if desired. If cooking the watercress, heat a non-stick frying pan over medium heat, add a teaspoon of water and the watercress, and briefly heat to wilt the watercress. Remove from the pan, drain and set aside.

In a bowl, mix together the eggs and water. Briefly scramble the eggs in the pan, stirring almost constantly for 1–2 minutes. Do not let it overcook — remove from the heat before the egg begins to brown around the edges. Season with quality sea salt if desired.

Lunch and dinner

Spiced Sweet Potato Soup

SERVES 4; PREPARATION TIME 15 MINUTES, COOKING TIME 35 MINUTES

This easy-to-prepare soup is rich in skin-loving minerals and it tastes absolutely lovely. The secret ingredient is Thai red curry paste (V+Vn, this ingredient may contain shrimp paste: see notes).

1½ tablespoons Thai red curry paste (V+Vn: 1 teaspoon yellow curry powder)

3 cups Anti-ageing Broth (p. 176, or use water)

3 cups filtered water

1 large organic vegetable stock cube

1 large red onion, peeled and diced

2 cloves garlic, minced

¼ cup dried red lentils

4 medium–large sweet potatoes, peeled and diced

In a large saucepan over medium heat, briefly sauté the curry paste/powder until fragrant (do not let the spices burn and add a splash of water if necessary). Add the broth, water, stock cube, onion and garlic and increase the heat to bring to the boil.

Meanwhile, prepare the dried lentils by rinsing them thoroughly in a large bowl of water, drain them and remove any discoloured ones. Add to the saucepan along with the sweet potato and stir to combine. Return to the boil, then reduce heat to low and simmer for 30 minutes. Remove the saucepan from the heat and allow to cool for 5 minutes.

Using a blender or food processor, blend the soup in batches to make a smooth soup. If the soup is too thick add ½ cup of water.

NOTES

✼ If desired, top with chopped fresh herbs such as coriander (cilantro) or parsley and serve with spelt sourdough bread. Store leftover red curry paste in the freezer.

Anti-ageing Broth

MAKES 8 CUPS OF BROTH; PREPARATION TIME 10 MINUTES, COOKING TIME
6 HOURS; MAKE 1 DAY BEFORE USE

The secret to a therapeutic broth is the addition of a weak acid, such as apple cider
vinegar or lemon juice, to draw out the minerals from the bones during cooking.
This alkaline broth is rich in collagen, glycine, calcium and magnesium. It boosts
liver detoxification (so it can have a detox effect), and has anti-inflammatory
and immunity-boosting ingredients. Use this broth during the 3-day Alkalising
Cleanse or as a tasty stock in casseroles and soups. (V+Vn: see notes.)

2 large beef bones, with a little meat on them (incl. necks, joints, marrow, lamb bones)

3.5 litres (7 ½pt) filtered water (room temperature, not heated)

1 large or 2 small free range/organic chicken carcasses

2 teaspoons apple cider vinegar or lemon juice

2 red onions

1 carrot

2 brussels sprouts

2 sticks celery

1 potato (use skins if not going green)

3–4 cloves garlic, minced

1 teaspoon Celtic sea salt (or quality sea salt)

Place the beef bones into a stockpot or very large saucepan along with the water,
chicken bones and apple cider vinegar or lemon juice. Cover, bring to the boil and
then simmer over low heat (do not add the vegetables yet). Meanwhile, wash,
scrub and chop the vegies into small pieces.

After about 2 hours of cooking, break apart the carcasses using tongs, to allow
more of the minerals to be extracted from the bones. Add the chopped vegetables
and the remaining ingredients. Cook for a total of 6 hours. The broth is more
flavoursome if it reduces almost by half.

Remove the larger bones using tongs (the chicken bones should crumble when
squeezed as the acid has caused the alkaline minerals to be extracted). Place a

strainer over a large bowl then pour the broth through the strainer. You can use a measuring cup to press down on the cooked meat and vegetables to squeeze out the remaining liquid. Discard the remaining bones and vegetables.

The next step is important: store the broth in a sealed container in the refrigerator overnight so the fat has time to solidify. The next day, carefully lift or skim off the layer of saturated fat and discard it.

NOTES

❇ V+Vn option: omit the bones and add extra vegetables and reduce cooking time to 3 hours; or use organic vegetable stock in the recipes.

❇ If your broth is thick and jelly-like, it means it's rich in collagen.

❇ Don't add purple vegetables to the stock or you'll end up with a purple broth.

❇ Broth will last for a week if refrigerated.

❇ Store the leftover broth in clean glass jars or containers and freeze the leftovers. Most soup/casserole recipes in this book use 3 cups of broth so measure out portions of 3 cups each and write the volume on the container before freezing.

Shiitake Vegetable Soup

SERVES 4; PREPARATION TIME 15 MINUTES, COOKING TIME 15 MINUTES

Shiitake mushrooms are rich in antioxidants, including selenium and vitamins A, E, C and vitamin D. They have been used as a medicinal food for centuries and are well known for their anti-tumour properties and for lowering blood pressure, strengthening the immune system against viruses, and for improving liver function (which is important for healthy skin).

But if you don't like shiitake mushrooms, swap them for ½ cup of finely diced eggplant (aubergine) — another vegetable packed with antioxidants in its skin.

5 cups filtered water

3 cups Anti-ageing Broth (p. 176; V+Vn: use filtered water)

1 large organic vegetable stock cube

1 red onion, finely diced

2 stalks celery, finely chopped

1 carrot, diced

1 teaspoon freshly grated ginger

¼ cup sliced shiitake mushrooms

1 tablespoon finely chopped parsley

1 tablespoon fresh lemon juice

Place the water, the broth, stock cube, onion, celery, carrot and ginger into a stockpot or large saucepan, cover with a lid and bring to the boil. Reduce heat and simmer on low for 10 minutes.

If you are using dried shiitake mushrooms, soak them in a bowl of warm water according to packet instructions (approximately 5 minutes) before cooking, then drain. Add the shiitake mushrooms and simmer for 5 minutes or until the vegetables are soft. Remove from heat.

Stir through the parsley and lemon juice and serve.

NOTES

✸ Variations: omit the celery and onion and add ¼ cup finely diced eggplant (aubergine). Or add ¼ cup of basmati rice, red quinoa or barley — quinoa takes 20–25 minutes to cook, or simmer the barley in a separate pot of water for 25 minutes if presoaked overnight (or 45 minutes if not soaked). Then add it to the soup (note: barley contains gluten).

Chicken and Barley Soup

SERVES 3; PREPARATION TIME 15 MINUTES, COOKING TIME 25 MINUTES
(OR 45 MINUTES IF BARLEY IS NOT PRE-SOAKED)

A delicious country-style chicken soup. Soak the barley overnight to reduce cooking time and increase mineral availability, or skip the soak and simply cook it for longer. Barley contains gluten so if you are gluten intolerant use basmati rice instead. (V+Vn: omit the chicken.)

¼ cup barley, rinsed (or use basmati rice)

2 chicken thigh fillets, skinless

½ lemon, juiced

6 cups (1.5L/3pt) filtered water

2 teaspoons organic vegetable stock or 2 vegetable stock cubes

1 red onion, finely diced (or celery)

1 carrot, diced

3 thin slices of eggplant (aubergine), finely diced

1 teaspoon freshly grated ginger

1 tablespoon finely chopped parsley

Place the barley in a saucepan of water and, if pre-soaked, simmer for 25 minutes (or 45 minutes if not pre-soaked). Drain and set aside. (If using basmati rice, cook it with the soup.) Dice the chicken and marinate it in the lemon juice for at least 10 minutes.

Place 6 cups of water, stock, onion, carrot, eggplant and ginger (and rice, if not using barley) into a stockpot or large saucepan, cover with a lid and bring to the boil. Reduce heat and simmer on low for 10 minutes.

Add the cooked barley, the chicken and 1 teaspoon of lemon juice from the marinade. Simmer for 5 minutes or until the chicken is cooked through (for tender chicken don't overcook). Remove from heat and stir through the parsley.

Beetroot and Carrot Salad

SERVES 4 AS A SIDE SALAD; PREPARATION TIME 10 MINUTES

Beetroot is rich in betaine which boosts the feel-good chemical serotonin in the brain, plus pigmented phytochemicals that protect DNA from damage. Here it's teamed with the goodness of lemon, apple and carrot.

3 medium carrots

2 large green apples, peeled

1 small fresh beetroot, top removed, washed and peeled

½ lemon, juiced

½ orange, juiced (approx. ¼ cup freshly squeezed orange juice)

handful of pomegranates seeds (or sultanas)

sprinkling of black sesame seeds

Using a large grater or a food processor, grate the carrots, apples and beetroot. Transfer to a non-metal bowl. Add the lemon juice, orange juice and pomegranate seeds and toss until well combined. Just before serving, sprinkle with black sesame seeds.

atercress Soup

SERVES 4; PREPARATION TIME 10 MINUTES, COOKING TIME 15 MINUTES

Watercress is highly alkalising and rich in calcium and hummus dip adds protein and a creamy texture with a hint of tang. When choosing potatoes, favour carisma or new potatoes as they have a lower GI than other varieties (avoid high GI varieties desiree, sebago, pontiac and nardine).

1–2 dollops Hummus Dip (p. 153; or store-bought hummus)

1 teaspoon garam masala

1 teaspoon freshly grated ginger

6 cups filtered water

2 heaped teaspoons organic vegetable stock

2 potatoes, peeled and diced

1 red onion, diced

1 bunch (140g/5oz) watercress, stalks trimmed 5cm (2in) (reserve 4 sprigs for garnish)

1 tablespoon fresh lemon juice

Prepare the hummus dip, if using, and set aside.

In a large saucepan over medium heat, lightly sauté the garam masala and ginger until fragrant (about 1 minute; do not let the spices burn). Place the water and stock into the saucepan and bring to the boil. Add the potato and onion and cover with a lid and simmer for 10 minutes.

Add the watercress and cook for 3–4 minutes. Then remove from heat and allow to cool for 5 minutes.

Add the lemon juice to the soup, then transfer to a blender or food processor and blend until smooth.

When serving, add a dollop of hummus dip (approx. 1½ teaspoons) to each bowl and mix slightly to give a creamy, streaked texture. Add another dollop of hummus to the centre of the soup and top with a sprig of watercress.

NOTES

* If you prefer, you can replace the 3 cups of water with 3 cups Anti-ageing Broth (p. 176).
* Serving suggestion: after the soup is served into bowls, sprinkle with a little sweet paprika and a sprig of watercress for presentation.

Parcel Baked Fish

SERVES 2; PREPARATION TIME 15 MINUTES, COOKING TIME 15 MINUTES

This Thai-styled fish dish is rich in omega-3 and the parcel baking method minimises AGEs during cooking. Serve it with steamed greens, such as green beans, broccolini and asparagus.

Coconut and Lime Marinade (p. 152; or marinade of choice)
1 or 2 fillets salmon or trout (see notes), skinless and boneless, halved lengthways
1 medium–large sweet potato, peeled and diced
¼ cup organic soy milk
freshly ground black pepper
1 small red chilli, sliced (or chilli flakes), optional
¼ cup coriander (cilantro) leaves

Make your marinade of choice and pour it over the fish and place it in the refrigerator until needed.

Preheat the oven to 160°C (320°F). In a small saucepan, bring some water to the boil, then boil or steam the sweet potato for 10–15 minutes or until very soft. Strain and return the sweet potato to the saucepan. Mash until lump-free, then stir in soy milk and pepper (if using) to make a creamy mash. Keep the mixture warm in the saucepan.

Cut two 30cm (12in) long sheets of baking paper. Place one into a high-sided baking dish and place one fish fillet onto it. Fold up the sides so the marinade does not spill when added, and repeat the process with the other fillet.

Top each fillet with chilli and spoon on some extra marinade (2 tablespoons will do). Close each parcel by sharply folding over the paper ends several times. Bake for 10–15 minutes, depending on thickness of the fish. *Tip:* slightly undercooking the fish keeps it lovely and tender. If you would like to cook the fish for longer, keep the parcels open and cook for another 2 minutes, then check again. Remove from heat.

Meanwhile, steam the greens for 3 minutes — they should remain crisp and bright green. Remove from the heat and uncover.

Open the fish parcels and place on plates, drizzle on a little of the cooked marinade and top with fresh coriander. Serve with the sweet potato mash.

NOTES

❀ Each serving size of fish should be around the size of the palm of your hand. Fish is usually sold in large pieces so you will probably only need half of one fillet per adult.

❀ Variations: top the fish with lime zest before cooking. Use another marinade such as Peach, Thyme and Chilli Marinade (p. 150).

❀ If fish develops white clumps on the sides, it is overcooked.

Sushi Rolls with Black Sesame

SERVES 2; PREPARATION TIME 25 MINUTES, COOKING TIME 20 MINUTES

Sushi is low GI, low in AGEs and rich in antioxidants and vitamin D. I recommend buying sushi mats to help you roll them to perfection. Raw salmon can be substituted with chicken, tofu or canned tuna.

1 cup sushi rice

1½ cups cold water

1 tablespoon apple cider vinegar

6 sheets nori (seaweed)

3 teaspoons black sesame seeds

Choose from the following fillings:

150–200g (5–7oz) sashimi-quality salmon (must be fresh)

½ avocado, sliced

red leaf lettuce, chopped (or mixed lettuce)

1 small cucumber

½ red capsicum (pepper), thinly sliced

Condiments:

wasabi (optional but should be used if eating raw fish)

tamari (or quality salt-reduced soy sauce)

pickled ginger (optional)

Place the rice and water into a saucepan and bring to the boil. Reduce heat to lowest setting, cover with a lid and simmer for 15 minutes. Add extra water if necessary, a little at a time. Turn the heat off but keep the rice on the stovetop for another 5 minutes. The rice should absorb all the water and be soft and sticky. Stir in the vinegar while the rice is hot then transfer to a bowl.

A sushi mat is not essential but it makes it much easier to form a perfect roll so if you have one you can use it. If not using a mat: place a nori sheet, shiny side down, onto a large plate or chopping board. Place a bowl of water within reach. Spoon some rice onto the nori. Wet your fingers then firmly pat down the rice to form a thin, even layer, leaving 2cm (⅘in) of nori uncovered at the end. Sprinkle the rice with approximately ½ teaspoon of black sesame seeds then add your filling of choice in a line (such as 3 slices of avocado and 3 thin slices of salmon).

Wet the exposed end of the nori sheet and begin carefully and tightly rolling from the opposite end. You can use a table knife to help you do this, placing the knife lengthways across the rice. The wet end should stick firmly. If using a mat: pick up the edges of the bamboo mat and tightly roll the sushi into cylinders. Then gently squeeze the mat to slightly compact the rice and hold it together. Using a very sharp knife dipped in water, cut each roll in half or, alternatively, into 2½cm (1in) pieces.

Serve with condiments — in a small bowl, mix a little hot wasabi (begin with the size of a pea) with 1–2 tablespoons of tamari. Pickled ginger can be placed on each plate.

Guava and Rocket Salad

SERVES 2; PREPARATION TIME 10 MINUTES

This tasty vegetarian meal is rich in protein, fibre, flavonoids and vitamin C. If available, use 2 small red guavas, or substitute with ½ large apple guava. Do not refrigerate guava as it tastes ripe and delicious at room temperature. If guava is unavailable use fresh figs or ½ cup pomegranate seeds. Serve on its own or with marinated chicken or Parcel Baked Fish (p. 184).

3 cups rocket (arugula) leaves (or mixed)

2 spring onions (scallions, shallots), green parts chopped diagonally

1 tablespoon Halo Dressing (p. 154)

½ avocado, sliced

4 small Kumatoes, sliced in half (see notes)

2 guavas, washed, de-seeded and sliced

½ teaspoon black sesame seeds

Wash and dry the rocket leaves using a salad spinner. Place in a salad bowl and add the spring onions.

Prepare the dressing, then add to the salad and lightly toss. Top with avocado, Kumatoes, guava and sprinkle with black sesame seeds.

NOTES

✿ If Kumatoes are not available in your area, substitute with roma (plum), vine-ripened or grape tomatoes.

Eggplant and Cauliflower Curry

SERVES 2; PREPARATION TIME 10 MINUTES, COOKING TIME 15 MINUTES

This tasty vegetarian curry is rich in cancer-protective flavonoids, enhanced by the addition of black pepper. The curry spices, cauliflower and ginger enhance phase II liver detoxification (elimination of chemicals and hormones), boost immunity and promote acid–alkaline balance in the body. The eggplant is rich in collagen-protective anthocyanins.

3 teaspoons mild yellow curry powder

1 teaspoon garam masala

½ teaspoon ground cinnamon

2 cloves garlic, minced

2½ cups organic vegetable stock or Anti-ageing Broth (p. 176)

1 cup finely diced eggplant (aubergine)

1½ teaspoons freshly grated ginger

1½ cups chopped cauliflower

½ cup coconut milk

½ cup basmati rice

1 cup loosely packed coriander (cilantro) leaves, chopped

ground black pepper

Heat a large saucepan over low heat and sauté the curry powder, garam masala, cinnamon and garlic for less than 1 minute. Add the stock or broth and bring to the boil. Add the eggplant, ginger, cauliflower and coconut milk, then reduce heat to a simmer for 15 minutes, stirring occasionally.

In another saucepan, bring plenty of water to the boil and cook the rice according to packet instructions (approx. 10 minutes). Drain.

Mix coriander into the curry.

Serve the curry on a bed of rice. Add pepper and garnish with extra coriander.

Winter Spiced Dahl

SERVES 2; PREPARATION TIME 10 MINUTES, COOKING TIME 22 MINUTES

This gluten-free vegetarian meal contains detoxifying spices and turmeric, which is rich in anti-cancer flavonoids, and the addition of black pepper enhances the protective effect.

1½ cups dried red lentils

1 large red onion, finely chopped

2 cloves garlic, minced

2 teaspoons yellow curry powder (mild or medium heat)

½ teaspoon ground cinnamon

1 teaspoon garam masala

2 cups filtered water

1 organic vegetable stock cube

5cm (2in) strip of kombu (seaweed)

1 cup loosely packed coriander (cilantro) leaves, chopped

ground black pepper

Soak the lentils in plenty of water and set aside.

Heat a large saucepan over medium heat, add the onion, garlic and a teaspoon of water and sauté briefly for 1 minute. Reduce the heat to low and add the curry powder, cinnamon and garam masala and sauté for 1 minute.

Drain the lentils and discard any that are discoloured. Add the lentils, water, stock cube and kombu to the saucepan and bring to the boil. Reduce the heat and simmer for 20 minutes. Break up the kombu and stir occasionally until lentils are soft and the dahl is smooth in consistency (it should not be runny or dry — add a touch more water if needed).

Stir through most of the coriander and add the pepper. Serve the dahl garnished with the remaining coriander.

NOTES

✳ Variations: serve with Curry Naan Bread, p. 193 (do not eat bread during the 3-day cleanse); if you can't eat onions substitute with 4 stalks of celery, finely diced. Use parsley instead of coriander; or add a squeeze of lemon and grated fresh ginger.

Spelt Flat Bread

MAKES 4 LARGE WRAPS (APPROX. 23CM/9IN EACH);
PREPARATION TIME 15 MINUTES, COOKING TIME 15 MINUTES

Making your own bread has a satisfying feeling, as if it's somehow good for the soul. This recipe is a simple one, with added cinnamon to keep blood sugar levels steady and to protect against AGE formation during cooking. It's wonderful for making salad wraps and can even be used as a pizza base — cheese-free pizza is easy to make and the recipe is on p. 194. This recipe also forms the basis for Curry Naan Bread (see notes).

1¼ cups plain spelt flour (preferably wholemeal), plus extra

1 teaspoon finely ground sea salt

¼ teaspoon ground cinnamon

¼ teaspoon bicarbonate of soda (baking soda)

1 tablespoon rice bran oil (see notes)

⅔ cup boiling water

In a bowl, mix the flour, salt, cinnamon and bicarb (sift together if necessary). Add the oil and the hot water and mix using a knife. Depending on the type of flour used, you may need more or less water — the dough should not be too stiff or sticky during the kneading process.

Lightly flour your chopping board and turn out the dough. Knead the dough for approximately 3 minutes until smooth and elastic, then cut into 4 balls. Place onto a plate, cover with plastic wrap and rest for 30 minutes on the kitchen bench (this is optional; you can cook them straightaway if necessary).

Again, lightly flour your chopping board (if making Curry Naan Bread add the curry powder now — see notes), then one by one roll each ball with a rolling pin to make large, thin circles (make them as thin as possible). Re-flour the board as necessary.

Heat a large non-stick frying pan over medium–high heat and briefly cook each flat bread for less than 1 minute each side or until bubbles appear. Pop bubbles as they appear so they don't become browned, and don't overcook them as the bread needs to stay soft. *Tip:* the bread should lighten all over as it's cooking.

NOTES

❀ If you have acne or oily skin use extra virgin olive oil instead of rice bran oil.

❀ Variation: add ¼ teaspoon of ground coriander (cilantro) or curry powder to increase protection from AGE formation or make Curry Naan Bread.

Curry Naan Bread

Follow the Spelt Flat Bread recipe and, where instructed, sprinkle some curry powder onto the chopping board, mix it with a little spelt flour and evenly coat the board. Then roll out your flat bread. Repeat the curry and flour process with each wrap.

Lemon Thyme Pizza

SERVES 2–4; PREPARATION TIME 20 MINUTES, COOKING TIME 20 MINUTES — IF YOU ARE MAKING THE PIZZA BASES ADD 15 MINUTES TO THE PREPARATION TIME

A lovely cheese-free pizza with chicken and fresh lemon thyme, an aromatic and therapeutic herb that contains antioxidants and has anti-inflammatory, antibacterial and antifungal activity thanks to thymol. Thyme leaves also protect and increase the beneficial fats in cell membranes. You have two chicken pizzas to choose from or make them prawn, vegetable or tofu if desired. Serve these with a side salad. If having without accompaniment, you may need 1½ or 2 pizzas per person. Use tomato paste in satchels or other preservative-free tomato pastes.

VERSION 1: CHICKEN AND TOMATO

2–4 Spelt Flat Bread (p. 192)

Anchovy and Mustard Marinade (p. 155)

3 skinless chicken thigh fillets, sliced and fat removed

2 satchels (100g/3½oz) tomato paste (preservative-fee)

2 vine-ripened tomatoes or 4 Kumatoes

½ cup fresh lemon thyme sprigs

Make the Spelt Flat Bread if not already made.

Make the marinade and mix most of it with the chicken pieces (reserve 1 tablespoon of marinade for the pizza). In a non-stick frying pan, lightly fry the chicken on medium heat until just cooked through (chicken should not be pink inside) — the mustard seeds will pop everywhere so you may need to use a lid.

Pre-heat the oven to 170°C (340°F). Line a baking tray with baking paper and place the spelt flat breads onto the tray. Spread with tomato paste (use about 25g/⅞oz for each base) and top with thin slices of tomato, chicken and a generous sprinkle of lemon thyme leaves. Place into the oven and bake for 5 minutes or until cooked to your liking.

Remove from oven and cut into slices. Top with plenty of fresh lemon thyme sprigs, about 2 sprigs per slice

VERSION 2: CHICKEN AND ZUCCHINI

2–4 Spelt Flat Bread (p. 192)

Peach, Thyme and Chilli Marinade (p. 150)

3 skinless chicken thigh fillets, sliced and fat removed

1 or 2 satchels (approx. 100g/3½oz) tomato paste (preservative-fee)

1 small zucchini (courgette), scrubbed

½ cup fresh lemon thyme sprigs

Make the Spelt Flat Bread if not already made.

Make the marinade and mix most of it with the chicken pieces (reserve 1 tablespoon of marinade for the pizza). In a non-stick frying pan, lightly fry the chicken on medium–high heat until just cooked through (chicken should not be pink inside). Remove from heat.

Pre-heat the oven to 170°C (340°F) and line a baking tray with baking paper. Place the spelt flat breads onto the baking tray. Spread the flat bread with tomato paste (use about 25g/¾oz for each base). Cut the zucchini into thin diagonal slices and add them to the pizza (don't crowd the pizza). If you have spare marinade, brush a little onto the zucchini slices. Add the chicken pieces and top with a generous sprinkle of lemon thyme leaves.

Bake the pizzas for 5 minutes then remove from oven and cut into slices. Top with plenty of fresh lemon thyme sprigs, about 2 sprigs per slice.

NOTES

❀ Variations: use white potato slices or roasted sweet potato, brushed with garlic oil, and steamed asparagus (steamed only for a minute or two). Or after cooking, top the middle of the pizzas with baby rocket (arugula) and a sprinkle of black pepper.

How to bake a sweet potato

1 sweet potato

½ teaspoon rice bran oil or extra virgin olive oil

a squeeze of lemon juice

Pre-heat the oven to 170°C (340°F) and line a baking tray with baking paper. Scrub the sweet potato and slice in half lengthways. Mix the oil and lemon juice and rub or brush it onto all surfaces of the sweet potato. Bake for 30 minutes or until soft all the way through.

Tip: cook extra sweet potato for use in Mixed Salad Wrap (p. 197) or pizza.

Mixed Salad Wrap

MAKES 1 WRAP; PREPARATION TIME 10 MINUTES (30 MINUTES COOKING TIME IF MAKING THE SPELT FLAT BREAD AND COOKING THE SWEET POTATO)

A healthy wrap rich in anthocyanins from the purple lettuce leaves and Kumatoes.

This is quite a large wrap but if you have a healthy appetite double the recipe.

1 Spelt Flat Bread (p. 192)

¼ large avocado

1 teaspoon lemon juice

4 slices roasted sweet potato (optional, if using leftovers)

1 cup mixed salad leaves

1 small spring onion (scallion, shallot), chopped

45g (1½oz) quality canned chunky tuna or Hummus Dip (p. 153; V+Vn option)

Optional toppings:

2 Kumatoes, chopped (see notes)

fresh coriander (cilantro), chopped

½ carrot, peeled and grated

Make the Spelt Flat Bread and bake the sweet potato (p. 196).

Mash the avocado and stir in the lemon juice. Then spread it onto the wrap.

In a strip, place onto the wrap the sweet potato, salad leaves, spring onion and tuna or hummus. If desired, add one or two optional toppings, then roll up the wrap.

NOTES

✻ If Kumatoes are not available in your area, substitute with roma (plum), vine-ripened or grape tomatoes.

Moroccan Lemon Chicken

SERVES 2; PREPARATION TIME 15 MINUTES, COOKING TIME 15 MINUTES

This antioxidant-rich curry has a mild, sweet flavour. The turmeric, lemon and ginger enhance liver detoxification (elimination of chemicals and hormones), boost immunity and promote acid–alkaline balance in the body.

400g (14oz) skinless chicken thigh fillets (approx. 3 large)

1 lemon

2 teaspoons yellow curry powder (mild or medium heat)

2 teaspoons garam masala

2 teaspoons brown rice flour (or spelt flour)

1 large red onion, roughly chopped

1 teaspoon freshly grated ginger

3 cups (750ml/1½pt) filtered water

1 organic vegetable stock cube (or powder)

½ cup basmati rice (¼ cup per person)

½ cup gourmet/Sicilian green olives

1 cup loosely packed coriander (cilantro) leaves, chopped

Slice the chicken into 1cm (½in) pieces and remove the fat. Juice half of the lemon and combine with the chicken (*don't marinate for more than 10 minutes or the lemon juice will start to 'cook' the chicken*). Cut the remaining lemon into four wedges and set aside.

Place the curry powder, garam masala and rice flour into a sealable bag and mix together. Remove the chicken and drain off the excess lemon and place the chicken into the bag. Seal it and shake to coat the chicken with the flour and spices.

Heat a large non-stick saucepan or wok over medium heat and sauté the onion until soft. Add the spiced chicken and fresh ginger and cook for 1 minute, enough to make the spices aromatic (do not burn them).

Add the water, vegetable stock and two of the lemon wedges to the pan, cover with a lid and bring to the boil. Reduce heat to low and simmer for 10 minutes or until the chicken is cooked through.

Meanwhile, boil the rice in a small saucepan of water for 10 minutes. Drain and set aside.

Add the olives to the pan and briefly heat for 1 minute. Remove from the heat and stir in the coriander. To serve, top with extra coriander and a fresh lemon wedge on each plate.

NOTES

❄ V+Vn: use firm tofu (not fried) instead of chicken or add green beans.

Sweet Potato Salad

SERVES 2; PREPARATION TIME 6 MINUTES, COOKING TIME 30 MINUTES

This is not an old-fashioned potato salad; the sweet potato stays whole while it's baked to perfection. It's lovely on its own but you can add some canned tuna or raw almonds for protein and variety, or serve with Oregano Chicken Sticks (p. 208). Make two serves so you can have tomorrow's lunch ready to go.

1 teaspoon lemon juice

1 teaspoon rice bran oil (see notes)

2 small sweet potatoes, skin scrubbed

quality sea salt

1 sprig fresh rosemary or lemon thyme (optional)

Avocado and Thyme Dip (p. 155) or dip of choice (see pp. 153–157 for options)

4 handfuls mixed salad leaves, washed

1 wedge of fresh lime

2 Kumatoes, sliced (or vine-ripened tomatoes)

black sesame seeds (optional)

Preheat the oven to 170°C (340°F). Line a baking tray with baking paper.

Mix the lemon juice with the oil and rub or brush some onto the sweet potatoes. Sprinkle with salt and top with fresh herbs and bake for 30 minutes or until you can easily pierce them with a fork. (If you want to speed up cooking time, cut sweet potatoes in half lengthways.)

Meanwhile, make the dip if not already prepared.

Remove the sweet potatoes from the oven. Halve lengthways and open them like a hot dog bun (if not already cut in half). Place the sweet potato onto serving plates and place the salad leaves to the side. Squeeze a little lime juice over both the potato and salad. Top the sweet potatoes with Kumatoes and dollop the salad with dip. Sprinkle over the black sesame seeds, if using.

NOTES

✵ Variation: add a little Anchovy and Mustard Dressing (p. 155) or a few
dollops of Beetroot and Almond Dip (p. 156) instead of the Avocado and
Thyme Dip.

✵ If you have oily or blemish-prone skin, avoid rice bran oil and use extra
virgin olive oil.

Shiitake Vegetable Casserole

SERVES 2; PREPARATION TIME 15 MINUTES, COOKING TIME 15 MINUTES

This soupy vegetarian casserole is rich in antioxidants including selenium and vitamins C, D and E. Shiitake mushrooms are well known for their anti-tumour properties and for lowering blood pressure, strengthening the immune system against viruses and for improving liver function, which is essential for healthy skin. If you don't like mushrooms, swap them for ½ cup of finely diced eggplant (aubergine) as they're rich in skin-protective anthocyanins.

2 cups chopped cauliflower

½ cup sliced shiitake mushrooms

½ cup finely diced red cabbage

1 tablespoon brown rice flour

2½ cups boiling filtered water, plus extra cool water

1 large organic vegetable stock cube

2 cloves garlic, minced

sprinkle of dried oregano or fresh lemon thyme

sprinkle of ground cinnamon

¼ cup fresh parsley leaves, finely chopped

Preheat the oven to 170°C (340°F). Place cauliflower, mushrooms and cabbage in large casserole dish and set aside.

In a large bowl, blend the flour with ¼ cup (60 ml/2fl oz) of *cool* water until smooth. Add the boiling water, stock cube and the garlic, mix well. Pour this over the vegetables. Sprinkle with oregano and cinnamon, then cover with a lid and place in the oven. Bake for 15 minutes or until the vegetables are tender but not overcooked.

Remove from the oven and stir through the parsley.

Quinoa and Pomegranate Salad

SERVES 2 (OR 4 AS A SIDE DISH); PREPARATION TIME 20 MINUTES

This antioxidant-rich salad is a classic dinner party dish, with a delicate balance of flavours. It is acid–alkaline balanced and the red quinoa contains anthocyanins and has a lower GI than the white variety.

1 cup red quinoa, rinsed

1 organic vegetable stock cube

1 large pomegranate

¼ teaspoon ground cinnamon

1 large lime, juiced (approx. 3 tablespoons)

1 teaspoon extra virgin olive oil

½ cup raw almonds, chopped (see notes)

1 cup mint leaves, finely chopped

Place the quinoa into a saucepan with 2½ cups water, cover and bring to the boil. Crumble in the stock cube and simmer on low heat for approximately 20 minutes or until the grains have softened (you should see plenty of white).

Meanwhile, remove the seeds from the pomegranate (see instructions on p. 204). Remove any discoloured ones. You will need about 1 cup of pomegranate seeds.

Drain the quinoa, sprinkle with the cinnamon and allow to cool. Then sprinkle on the lime juice and olive oil and mix.

Add the pomegranate seeds, chopped almonds and mint to the salad and lightly toss. Add extra lime juice to taste, if necessary.

NOTES

❀ Variation: use ½ cup of mint leaves and ½ cup of chopped coriander (cilantro) leaves and top with black sesame seeds.

❀ If you have oily or blemish-prone skin avoid almonds and use no nuts or use lightly toasted pine nuts instead.

❀ Black quinoa: this recipe does not work with black quinoa as it does not soak up liquid well. If you cannot find red quinoa use white quinoa, which takes 15–20 minutes to cook.

How to choose and de-seed a pomegranate

When shopping for a pomegranate, choose a nice heavy one that has firm, unwrinkled skin with no decaying or softened patches. The easy way to de-seed a pomegranate involves submerging it in water — this prevents everything from staining red and the seeds sink to the bottom, while the white pith floats to the top. *Tip:* make your cuts shallow so you don't damage the seeds.

1. Place the pomegranate in a bowl of water.

2. Using a sharp knife, cut the top off the pomegranate. You can do this in one long shallow cut about ½cm (⅛in) deep, following the outer ridge at the top. Or you can do this in four cuts, like a square lid.

3. Lift the lid off the pomegranate and remove any seeds attached to the lid and place them in the water.

4. Note the wedge formations inside the pomegranate caused by the white pith. Shallow cut the skin of the pomegranate following the natural wedge lines — there will be about five wedges, depending on the size of your pomegranate.

5. Break the wedges apart and gently remove the seeds while in the water. Throw out as much pith as possible and let the rest float to the top.

6. Scoop out the floating pith and discard any damaged, discoloured or whitish seeds, then strain the remaining seeds and drain well.

Mango and Black Sesame Salad

SERVES 2 AS A SIDE SALAD; PREPARATION TIME 10 MINUTES

3 cups mixed baby salad leaves, washed and dried

4 small Kumatoes, halved (see notes)

½ ripe avocado sliced

1 quality mango, diced

1 tablespoon Halo Dressing (p. 154; see notes)

1 teaspoon black sesame seeds

Arrange the salad leaves on a platter and dot with Kumatoes. Add the sliced avocado and mango and drizzle on the dressing. Sprinkle on the black sesame seeds.

NOTES

❀ If Kumatoes are not available in your area, substitute with roma (plum), vine-ripened or grape tomatoes.

❀ If you have oily or blemish-prone skin omit the salad dressing and use a squeeze of fresh lime juice instead.

How to tell if an avocado is ripe (before you buy)

Gently press on the tip of the avocado. If it is soft it's ripe but if the whole avocado is soft it may be overripe and starting to bruise.

Mediterranean Seafood Soup

SERVES 2; PREPARATION TIME 20 MINUTES, COOKING TIME 10 MINUTES

A lovely flavoursome soup that requires flathead. If flathead is not available use any low mercury fish such as salmon or trout (see p. 68 for the fish list). You can also use 400g (14oz) of quality seafood marinara mix *if it does not contain basa* or high mercury fish (see p. 69 for list). The bean sprouts and lemon are important alkalising ingredients that give this meal acid–alkaline balance.

3 large roma (plum) tomatoes (whole, must have no cuts)

1 large red onion, halved and finely diced

1½ teaspoons smoked paprika

1 teaspoon cumin

2 garlic cloves, minced

3½ cups boiling filtered water

1 organic vegetable stock cube

1 fillet boneless flathead (approx 200g/7oz), cut into 2½cm (1in) pieces

6 green prawns, peeled and de-veined (see prawn tips, p. 207)

100g (3½oz) raw calamari rings (no breadcrumbs) or use calamari tube, sliced

½ lemon, juiced

½ cup bean sprouts, washed in water with a splash of vinegar

½ cup fresh coriander (cilantro) leaves, extra to garnish

Place the tomatoes into a small saucepan and cover with water. Bring to the boil and simmer for 5 minutes or until the skins split (*tip:* the skins won't split if the tomato has been cut). Remove the tomatoes from the saucepan and allow to cool slightly, then remove and discard the skins and hard core and slice. Mash the soft flesh until runny.

Meanwhile, heat a large saucepan over medium heat. Add the onion and about 1 tablespoon of water and sauté for a few minutes or until the onion softens. Reduce the heat and add the smoked paprika, cumin and garlic and cook, stirring, for less than 1 minute or until aromatic, being careful not to burn the spices. Add the mashed tomato, the water and crumble the stock cube into the water and bring to the boil.

Reduce the heat and simmer for 5 minutes. Then add the fish, prawns and calamari. Simmer for 5 minutes or until seafood is cooked to your liking (don't overcook).

Remove from the heat and add 1 tablespoon of lemon juice, or more if desired. Stir in the coriander. Top with the bean sprouts and use extra coriander for garnish.

NOTES

✿ Variations: add ¼ cup cooked quinoa (red or white) to the soup (cook it separately as it will take an extra 15 minutes) or add ¼ cup of basmati rice to the soup at the beginning of cooking. Zest the lemon and add to the soup or add ½ teaspoon freshly grated ginger.

How to peel and de-vein a whole prawn

Take off the head first by digging your thumbnail under one side of the head and removing the head.

Next, dig in your thumbnail at the underbelly side and unwrap the prawn shell from the meat, repeat until you reach the tail.

Dig your nail into the underside of the tail and split it, then gently remove the tail (some people like to leave the tail on for presentation and then remove them at the dinner table — it's up to you).

The easiest way to **de-vein the prawn** is to use a knife and make a very shallow cut running along one-third of the back of the prawn, from which the 'vein' can then be pulled out. Rinse the prawns if necessary.

Use prawns in Mediterranean Seafood Soup (p. 206) or pop them on skewers — you can follow the Oregano Chicken Sticks recipe (p. 208).

Note: raw prawns are often treated with sulfite preservative so avoid them if you are sensitive to sulfites. However, some *cooked* prawns are sulfite-free and your local fishmonger can advise on which ones these are.

Oregano Chicken Sticks

SERVES 2, PREPARATION TIME 25 MINUTES, COOKING TIME 20 MINUTES

This fun dish is not only ideal for chicken, it's also suitable for firm tofu, peeled prawns, salmon and other fresh fish fillets (see notes). You can also use other marinades such as Peach, Thyme and Chilli Marinade (p. 150).

Tamari, Lime and Ginger Marinade (p. 152)

3 large (approx. 400g/14oz) skinless chicken thigh fillets

½ cup red or white quinoa, rinsed (use more if desired)

1 organic vegetable stock cube

sprinkle of ground cinnamon

6–8 bamboo skewers

8 very small Kumatoes or grape tomatoes, halved

large oregano leaves

Celtic sea salt (optional)

8 asparagus spears, ends trimmed

2 large red cabbage leaves

Cut the chicken into cubes and trim the fat. Coat the chicken in the marinade and set aside in the refrigerator.

Meanwhile, fill a shallow baking tray with water and soak the bamboo skewers for at least 15 minutes to prevent them from burning during cooking.

Next, cook the quinoa (refer to 'How to cook quinoa' on p. 209) and set aside.

Remove the skewers from the water and take the chicken out of the fridge. Thread half a Kumato onto each skewer, leaving a 5cm (2in) space at the blunt end of the skewers. Then in alternating patterns, thread the chicken and the large oregano leaves onto the skewers (two chicken pieces to one oregano leaf) and end with another half Kumato. Season with salt.

Preheat the grill (broiler) to medium heat. Grill the chicken skewers for 10–15 minutes, turning once, or until thoroughly cooked (chicken must be cooked through but not overcooked so check frequently).

Fill a large saucepan with about 2½cm (1in) of boiling water. Place the asparagus and cabbage leaves into a steamer basket and steam for 2–3 minutes. Serve the asparagus and skewers onto serving plates and spoon the quiona into the cabbage cups.

NOTES

✹ You can make 'Fish on Sticks' by using salmon or trout and cook for approximately 5 minutes. They will cook quickly so be careful not to overcook.

How to cook quinoa

For a small side serve of quinoa for 2 people, you will need:

½ cup red quinoa, rinsed (use more if desired, or use white quinoa)

1 organic vegetable stock cube

sprinkle of ground cinnamon

Place the quinoa into a saucepan with 1½ cups of water and the crumbled stock cube, cover and bring to the boil. Simmer over low heat for approximately 20 minutes or until the grains have softened (if using red quinoa you should see plenty of white). Drain, and sprinkle with cinnamon to keep your blood sugar levels steady during consumption.

Steamed Chicken and Mint Meatballs

MAKES 28 MEATBALLS; PREPARATION TIME 15 MINUTES,
COOKING TIME 21 MINUTES

This healthy steamed meatballs recipe is easy to make and tastes great served with Ginger and Lime Dipping Sauce. You'll need a food processor to make the recipe quickly and easily. This recipe makes many meatballs so freeze the leftovers (see notes). Serve with salad or steamed green vegetables and quinoa (refer to 'How to cook quinoa' on p. 209).

½ red onion peeled and roughly chopped

600g (1⅓lb) skinless chicken thigh fillets

1 small bunch mint leaves, picked (more than ½ cup packed leaves)

½ cup coriander (cilantro) leaves

1 teaspoon mild yellow curry powder

1 teaspoon tamari

brown rice flour (or wholemeal spelt flour)

quality sea salt

ground black pepper

Ginger and Lime Dipping Sauce (p. 157; optional)

Place the onion into a food processor and process briefly until finely diced. Roughly chop the chicken, removing any fat, and add the chicken pieces to the processor. Process until the chicken becomes minced. Add the mint, coriander, curry powder and tamari and process until the ingredients stick together.

Cover a large plate with rice flour and sprinkle with salt and pepper. Using a tablespoon, scoop the chicken mixture and form into balls (approx. 4cm/1½in diameter), rolling them in the brown rice flour and dusting off the excess. Place the completed meatballs on another plate and continue until all the mixture has been used. *Tip:* you will eat approximately five each, so you can freeze the excess (separated by plastic wrap or baking paper in containers) and cook them as needed.

Place 5cm (2in) of water into a saucepan and bring to the boil. Place the meatballs in a steamer basket, in batches, then place the basket over the boiling water, cover with a lid and steam the meatballs on high heat for approximately 5–7 minutes (check the first batch to determine cooking time). Place the steamed meatballs onto paper towels to drain.

If steaming vegetables: briefly clean the steamer basket then steam greens such as peas, asparagus and broccolini for 3 minutes. Serve with the dipping sauce, if desired.

NOTES

❀ Leftover cooked meatballs can be used in Mixed Salad Wrap (p. 197).

Steamed Fish with Lime and Ginger

SERVES 2; PREPARATION TIME 15 MINUTES, COOKING TIME 15 MINUTES

2 cobs of corn

Coconut and Lime Marinade (p. 152)

2 (approx 350g/12oz) fillets boneless flathead (or similar low mercury fish)

Celtic sea salt (or other quality sea salt)

1 zucchini (courgette), ends trimmed (this will be peeled in long strips)

8 asparagus spears, ends trimmed

1 cup frozen peas

2–4 sprigs coriander (cilantro)

Place the corn into a saucepan and cover with water. Bring to the boil and simmer for 15 minutes then set aside.

Mix half of the marinade with the fish. Place some water into another saucepan, then place the fish in a steamer basket over the saucepan. Steam the fish for 5–7 minutes or until cooked to your liking. Heat the remaining marinade in a separate saucepan.

Steam the peas for 5 minutes and the asparagus for 3 minutes, then serve with the fish and corn. Garnish the fish with fresh coriander and serve the heated marinade as a sauce on the side.

Chapter 12

Shopping list

The following shopping list covers all the ingredients you'll need to follow the 28-day menu; amounts may vary, however, as some fresh and perishable items will need to be bought when needed and when in season (or choose seasonal alternatives). When shopping, choose products that are free of artificial additives (preservatives, colours, flavour enhancers). Remember, too, that fresh is best and if possible favour free range and organic products.

Fresh produce

PERISHABLE ITEMS, BUY THESE WEEKLY
OR AS NEEDED:

[ ] AVOCADOS*
[ ] BEETROOT
[ ] LEMONS*
[ ] LIMES*
[ ] MIXED SALAD LEAVES*
    (WITH PURPLE LEAVES)
[ ] PEACHES (2 FOR MARINADE)
[ ] PARSLEY
[ ] OREGANO LEAVES
[ ] LEMON THYME*
[ ] MINT
[ ] CORIANDER (CILANTRO)*
[ ] GINGER*
[ ] GARLIC
[ ] BANANA
[ ] GREEN APPLES
[ ] BLUEBERRIES*
[ ] FROZEN RASPBERRIES
[ ] PAPAYA
[ ] CHERRIES
[ ] GUAVA (PREF. RED)
[ ] POMEGRANATE
[ ] KUMATOES (OR ROMA/PLUM OR
    GRAPE TOMATOES)
[ ] SWEET POTATO*
[ ] BROCCOLI OR BROCCOLINI
[ ] CARROTS (ORANGE AND PURPLE)*
[ ] CELERY (FOR JUICING)
[ ] RED CAPSICUM (PEPPER)
[ ] CUCUMBER (FOR JUICING)
[ ] KALE (FOR JUICING)
[ ] MIXED SPROUTS
[ ] WATERCRESS
[ ] RED ONION*
[ ] SPRING ONIONS
    (SCALLIONS, SHALLOTS)

[ ] POTATO (FOR MAKING BROTH)
[ ] SHIITAKE MUSHROOMS (OR DRIED)
[ ] ¼ CAULIFLOWER
[ ] ¼ RED CABBAGE
[ ] ASPARAGUS
[ ] ZUCCHINI (COURGETTE)

Pantry items

[ ] SPELT FLOUR* (PREF. WHOLEMEAL)
[ ] BROWN RICE FLOUR
[ ] BICARBONATE OF SODA
    (BAKING SODA)
[ ] ROLLED OATS* (NOT INSTANT)
[ ] SUNRICE 'LOW GI' BROWN RICE
[ ] BASMATI RICE
[ ] RED QUINOA HF (IF UNAVAILABLE
    BUY WHITE)
[ ] RICE BRAN OIL*
[ ] EXTRA VIRGIN OLIVE OIL (FIRST
    COLD PRESSING)*
[ ] APPLE CIDER VINEGAR* HF
[ ] QUALITY SEA SALT (E.G. CELTIC OR
    MACRO HF)*
[ ] GROUND BLACK PEPPER
[ ] BLACK SESAME SEEDS HF
[ ] CANNED ANCHOVY FILLETS
[ ] RICE MALT SYRUP HF
[ ] YELLOW BOX HONEY OR
    ORGANIC HONEY
[ ] RAW ALMONDS (NOT SALTED OR
    ROASTED)
[ ] DRIED OR CANNED CHICKPEAS
[ ] CAROB POWDER
[ ] DANDELION ROOT TEA (OPTIONAL)
[ ] GINGER TEA BAGS (OPTIONAL)
[ ] CHAI TEA BAGS (OPTIONAL)
[ ] SUSHI RICE, NORI SHEETS
    (IF MAKING SUSHI)
[ ] SUSHI MAT, WASABI, GINGER
    (IF MAKING SUSHI)

[ ] DRIED RED LENTILS
[ ] KOMBU (FOR DAHL)
[ ] ORGANIC VEGETABLE STOCK
 CUBES* **HF** (E.G. SWISS NATURE)
[ ] TOMATO PASTE (SACHETS),
 PRESERVATIVE-FREE
[ ] 20 BAMBOO SKEWERS

Spices
[ ] GROUND CINNAMON*
 (PREF. CEYLON)
[ ] GARAM MASALA*
[ ] YELLOW CURRY POWDER*
[ ] GROUND CUMIN
[ ] SWEET PAPRIKA
[ ] SMOKED PAPRIKA
[ ] CHILLI FLAKES (OPTIONAL)
[ ] WHOLE CLOVES

Fridge/freezer
PERISHABLE ITEMS, BUY THESE WEEKLY
OR AS NEEDED:

[ ] LINSEEDS/FLAXSEEDS (WHOLE) **HF**
[ ] WHOLEGRAIN MUSTARD
[ ] TAMARI*
 (SALT-REDUCED) **HF**
[ ] ORGANIC TOMATO SAUCE
 (KETCHUP)
[ ] LIGHT COCONUT MILK
[ ] COCONUT WATER
[ ] TAHINI
 (HULLED TASTES BETTER) **HF**
[ ] ORGANIC FLAXSEED OIL
 (OPTIONAL) **HF**
[ ] SOY LECITHIN GRANULES,
 NON-GMO (OPTIONAL) **HF**
[ ] LIQUID CHLOROPHYLL
 (OPTIONAL) **HF**

[ ] EGGS **FRO** (OMEGA ENRICHED)
[ ] BONES FOR BROTH (2 BEEF, 1–2
 CHICKEN CARCASSES) **FRO**
[ ] CHICKEN THIGH FILLETS* **FRO**
[ ] FISH* (SALMON, TROUT, FLATHEAD)
[ ] PRAWNS
[ ] CALAMARI RINGS/TUBES
[ ] ORGANIC SOY MILK
 (FRESH IS BEST)
[ ] FROZEN PEAS

Guide to symbols

FRO = CHOOSE FREE RANGE OR
 ORGANIC WHERE POSSIBLE.
* DENOTES A 'HIGH-USE'
 INGREDIENT IF FOLLOWING
 THE 14-DAY MENU.
HF = AVAILABLE FROM THE
 HEALTH FOOD SECTION IN
 LARGE SUPERMARKETS OR
 HEALTH FOOD SHOPS.

Skin problem chart

Note: Before taking supplements refer to 'Health note' on p. 77 to see if supplementation is right for you.

Signs of skin ageing and other skin problems	Recommendations covered in this book	Other options not covered in this book
abscesses, skin ulcers, bacterial skin infections		see your doctor
acne	follow the 28-day program; *avoid* fried foods, red meat, dairy, sugar, almonds, flaxseeds/linseeds and cooking oils; change skin care products (as your current ones could be causing the problem); drink 8 glasses of filtered water daily; drink fresh vegetable juice; check for ʒinc or vitamin A deficiency; use anti-scar silicon sheets over healing acne to prevent scarring	for supplement advice speak to a naturopath or read the acne chapter in *The Healthy Skin Diet* (Exisle Publishing)
aged skin	follow the 28-day program; wear a hat and sunscreen (at least SPF30+ on the body and SPF50 on your face, neck, chest and hands); take a calcium and omega-3 supplement	a cosmetic physician or dermatologist can advise on other options
age spots (liver spots, sun spots, lentigines) on sun-exposed areas	use pigmentation fade/bleach creams such as John Plunkett; use AHA skin care (see p. 100); wear SPF50 sunscreen esp. on hands, face and chest to limit new ones appearing (SPF30 or less is not enough to prevent age spots)	a cosmetic physician or a dermatologist can advise on stronger treatment options such as laser treatment

Signs of skin ageing and other skin problems	Recommendations covered in this book	Other options not covered in this book
bruising, easy or with no apparent reason, purplish spots on skin	check for vitamin C deficiency (early scurvy sign)	see your doctor
bumpy skin or keratosis	follow the 28-day program; take an omega-3 fish oil supplement or flaxseed oil daily; avoid cigarette smoke; check for vitamin A, zinc or EFA deficiency (see p. 90)	see your doctor, nutritionist or a naturopath if symptoms persist
cellulite	follow the 28-day program; avoid dairy and alcohol; drink filtered water daily; do toning exercise and soft sand jogging; take a calcium supplement (p. 78)	
chest wrinkles after sleep	avoid drinking alcohol; apply body butter to area before and after sleep; use AHA and retinol in skin care; sleep flat on your back (p. 124); drink 8 glasses of filtered water daily; wear SPF50 sunscreen if exposing your décolletage to the sun	
dandruff	follow the 28-day program; change your shampoo (avoid SLS/sulfates in shampoo); try this recipe for Tea Tree Shampoo: add to your shampoo 1 teaspoon apple cider vinegar and ½ teaspoon tea tree oil, and shake. Shampoo daily until symptoms improve	take a probiotic supplement (containing Lactobacillus rhamnosus; L. rhamnosus GG; and/or L. acidophilus LA5)
dermatitis or contact dermatitis		avoid contact irritants and refer to The Eczema Diet (Exisle Publishing) for dietary and skin care advice

Signs of skin ageing and other skin problems	Recommendations covered in this book	Other options not covered in this book
dry skin	take a calcium supplement; follow the 28-day program; drink 8 glasses of filtered water daily; take an omega-3 fish oil supplement or flaxseed oil daily; use almonds and rice bran oil in cooking; avoid vitamin A oral supplements as they dry the skin; eat guava, papaya and other yellow foods; use suitable moisturisers	
eczema		refer to *The Eczema Diet* (Exisle Publishing) for dietary and skin care advice
enlarged pores and blackheads	follow the 28-day program; reduce fat and oil intake to reduce sebum production; take a zinc supplement (p. 234) and possibly vitamin A; use skin care products containing retinol and AHA (p. 100); they can take a long time to reduce naturally	a beautician, dermatologist or cosmetic physician can advise on other options
fungal infection on feet or nails, tinea		use tea tree oil topically; see your doctor, a pharmacist or a naturopath for stronger treatments
melasma (chloasma, hyper-pigmentation)	it may resolve on its own if caused by pregnancy; skin care products containing retinol and AHAs may marginally help such as John Plunkett (see p. 236); wear sunscreen with SPF50 on affected areas; home treatments may not be strong enough to remove all melasma	a cosmetic physician or a dermatologist can advise on other options

Signs of skin ageing and other skin problems	Recommendations covered in this book	Other options not covered in this book
menopause-related skin problems (dry and dull skin, reduced skin tone, poor skin immunity, wrinkles)	follow the 28-day program; take a chromium supplement (p. 81); 1200mg of calcium daily, plus magnesium, copper and vitamin D ('Calcium Complete', see p. 234); active skin care plus a hydrating moisturiser applied on top (Synergie have moisturisers for ageing skin); daily exercise.	see your doctor for frequent check-ups to rule out other causes
pallor (pale, unhealthy looking complexion)	improve blood flow to the skin with daily exercise; check for biotin deficiency; refer to nutrient deficiency questionnaire (p. 90); increase intake of alkalising foods to improve blood flow (refer to acid–alkaline food charts, starting on p. 226)	have a general check-up with your doctor to rule out other factors
hyper-pigmentation; mottled pigmentation	use fade/bleach creams containing AHA such as John Plunkett (see p. 236); wear SPF50 sunscreen on affected areas; home treatments may not be strong enough to remove all pigmentation (especially after pregnancy)	a cosmetic physician or a dermatologist can advise on other options
psoriasis	follow a fresh, healthy diet, avoid junk food; avoid cigarette smoke; learn to manage stress; no alcohol	use water, sunlight and oil therapy and liver cleansing (refer to the psoriasis chapter in *The Healthy Skin Diet*, Exisle Publishing)
rosacea	daily exercise is essential	limit histamine foods in the diet (refer to the rosacea chapter in *The Healthy Skin Diet*, Exisle Publishing)
rough skin	exfoliate (p. 111); take an omega-3 fish oil supplement (p. 84) or flaxseed oil daily; drink 8 glasses of filtered water daily; use skin care products containing AHAs (p. 100)	a beautician or a dermatologist can advise on other options

Signs of skin ageing and other skin problems	Recommendations covered in this book	Other options not covered in this book
sagging skin, age related, post-pregnancy or from weight loss	follow the 28-day program and increase protein in the diet if necessary; exercise and use weights daily (see a personal trainer for a program to suit your needs); check for nutritional deficiencies especially copper (p. 91) and ʒinc (p. 94) take 1000 to 1200mg of calcium daily ('Calcium Complete', p. 234)	a cosmetic physician can advise on other options
sensitive, dry skin	follow the 28-day program; take omega-3 fish oil (p. 84); avoid sulfites in skin care (p. 107); use gentle skin care	
slow wound healing	follow the 28-day program; check for nutritional deficiencies (p. 90)	see your doctor
spider veins and varicose veins	no natural way to reverse them but you can limit further damage and reduce pain by avoiding standing up on hard surfaces for extended periods and by reducing saturated fat intake — *avoid* eating red meat, pork and chicken skin	cosmetic physicians and vein specialists can effectively treat vein problems
stretch marks	can occur if you are ʒinc deficient during pregnancy or during weight gain (ʒinc deficiency signs listed on p. 94); it's hard to reverse but products containing retinol and AHAs may help (pp. 99–102); to avoid future problems: take a ʒinc supplement or eat ʒinc rich foods (p. 88) and vitamin C-rich foods (p. 80); moisturise your skin daily	a cosmetic physician or a dermatologist can advise on other options
uneven skin tone	follow the 28-day program; check for nutritional deficiencies (p. 90); do daily exercise; use skin care products containing retinol and AHA (p. 100); correct with make-up (p. 114)	a cosmetic physician, beautician or dermatologist can advise on other options

Signs of skin ageing and other skin problems	Recommendations covered in this book	Other options not covered in this book
wrinkles	follow the 28-day program to reduce appearance of fine lines; check for nutritional deficiencies (p. 90); take calcium (p. 234) and omega-3 (p. 84) or add flaxseeds/linseeds to your diet (p. 74); avoid future sun damage by wearing a hat and sunscreen (SPF50) daily to protect face, neck, hands and chest (even on cloudy days)	a cosmetic physician or dermatologist can advise on other options
yellow skin and eyes	follow the 28-day program and reduce AGEs in your diet; check for nutritional deficiencies — refer to nutrient deficiency questionnaire (p. 90); consuming large amounts of carrots can cause skin discolouration	see your doctor for a check-up to rule out other factors such as liver problems

AGE food list

The following table lists foods from lowest to highest amount of dietary AGEs contained. Your daily AGE consumption should not exceed 5000–8000 kilounits (kU). So if you consume 100g (3½oz) of anything in the 'very high' column on the right-hand side, you could exceed the recommended daily intake.

Tips

❄ Favour foods in the first two columns — 'low' and 'low–medium'.

❄ Avoid everything listed in the 'high' and 'very high' column.

The following table is based on AGE kU per 100g (3½oz), carboxymethyl-lysine (CLM) content only — other types of AGEs might be present).[1]

low-AGE foods: 0–99	low–medium AGE foods: 100–999	high AGE foods: 1000–4999	very high AGE foods: 5000+
apple	plums	chicken mince, fried	bacon
banana	raisins	lamb, marinated	butter
tomato	almonds, raw	veal, stewed	margarine
tomato sauce (ketchup)	avocado	crab meat, fried	mayonnaise
most fruits	pistachios	salmon, pan-fried	cream cheese
egg white	salad dressing	prawns, pan-fried	peanuts
omelette, low heat	scrambled eggs (high heat for 1 min)	cottage cheese	beef mince, fried
1 egg, poached	Greek bread	moʒʒarella, reduced fat	peanut butter
scrambled eggs (low heat for 2 mins)	granola	tofu, fried/grilled (broiled)	canola oil
wholemeal bread, untoasted	pasta	1 egg, fried	cottonseed oil

low-AGE foods: 0–99	low–medium AGE foods: 100–999	high AGE foods: 1000–4999	very high AGE foods: 5000+
bran flakes	chicken, poached with lemon	biscuits (cookies)	sesame oil
oatmeal	chicken, steamed with lemon	muesli (granola) bars	sausages
rolled oats	chicken (marinated with lemon)	dried figs	deli meats
porridge	fish loaf	almonds, blanched or roasted	frankfurter
rice	fish (steamed in foil with lemon)		beef hamburger
potatoes	canned salmon		roast beef
carrots	smoked salmon		pizza, store-bought
celery	raw trout or salmon		toasted cheese melt
cucumber	soy burger		steak, pan-fried
green beans	raw tofu		roasted chicken
onion	kidney beans		deep-fried chicken
most vegetables	coconut milk		chicken, fried in oil
mixed salad leaves	corned beef		chicken nuggets
vegetable juice	bagel		chicken kebab
veggie burger	grilled (broiled) eggplant (aubergine)		beef kebab
chicken soup	grilled (broiled) vegetables		most cheeses
vegetable soup	hummus, commercial		feta
lentil soup			
soy sauce			
tamari			
herbal tea			
black tea			

Swap this for that

Pioneering AGE researchers Dr Uribarri and Dr Vlassara recommend that your daily AGE consumption *should not exceed 5000–8000 kilounits*. However, the typical Western diet is very rich in AGEs and the average AGE consumption is approximately 15,000 and up to 25,000 kilounits daily (those who consumed more than 10,000 were found by the researchers to be prone to being overweight or had diabetes and other health problems).

The following tables list some typical food choices for meals throughout the day, along with AGE amounts; these are then followed by low-AGE alternatives.

Breakfast no. 1: high-AGE breakfast
THIS BREAKFAST WILL MAKE YOU EXCEED YOUR DAILY INTAKE OF AGES.

Food	AGE content
2 fried eggs (100g/3½oz)	2749
2 slices white toast (60g/2oz) with butter (10g/⅓oz)	2712
1 cup coffee (from pot of brewed coffee which has been on a heating plate for 1 hour)	34
Total AGEs:	**5495**

Breakfast no. 2: low-AGE breakfast

Food	AGE content
2 poached eggs* (100g/3½oz)	90
wholewheat toast, no butter or margarine (100g/3½oz)	120
1 bowl porridge	18
1 cup of tea	5
Total AGEs:	**233**

*2 eggs *scrambled on low heat* with minimal olive oil is also a good option, with 97 kU/100g

Lunch no. 1: high-AGE lunch

Food	AGE content
grilled chicken (100g/3½oz)	5200
2 slices of white bread (60g/2oz), with butter (10g/⅓oz)	2417
1 cup coffee (from pot of brewed coffee which has been on a heating plate for 1 hour)	34
Total AGEs:	**7651**

Lunch no. 2: low-AGE lunch

Food	AGE content
chicken, poached with lemon (100g/3½oz)	861
wholewheat bread, no butter or margarine (100g/3½oz)	53
1 cup mixed salad leaves	17
avocado, used as a spread (10g/ ⅓oz)	158
1 cup coffee	6
1 apple	15
Total AGEs:	**1110**

Dinner no. 1: high-AGE dinner

Food	AGE content
steak, pan-fried in oil (100g/3½oz)	10,058
homemade French fries (100g/3½oz)	694
1 cup of hot chocolate for dessert	656
Total AGEs:	**11,408**

Dinner no. 2: low-AGE dinner

Food	AGE content
salmon, poached or steamed (100g/3½oz)*	1477
grilled (broiled) vegetables (100g/3½oz)	226
rice (100g/3½oz)	9
1 banana for dessert (100g/3½oz)	9
Total AGEs:	**1721**

*no data showing AGE content if pre-marinated

Total daily AGEs for no. 1 = 24,554   Total daily AGEs for no. 2 = 3064

Acid–alkaline food charts

The following charts list alkalising and acidifying products. It also shows the main natural and artificial chemicals present for those who have sensitivities (refer to Symbols chart).

Symbols and abbreviations

(MSG)	natural or artificial flavour enhancer
(GI)	food with a high glycaemic index (use cinnamon with it!)
(G)	contains gluten
(P)	may contain preservatives and/or artificial sweetener/flavours/colours
Ω	good source of omega-3 (eat fish three times a week and flaxseed/linseed oil/seeds daily, if no allergy)

Beverages

Strongly alkalising	Alkalising	Acidifying	Strongly acidifying
green detox powder	Moisture Boost Smoothie, p. 164	beer	alcohol
vegetable juice, fresh	Almond Milk, p. 168	carob powder	black tea
Green Glow Juice, p. 162	herbal teas	fruit juice	cocoa, hot chocolate (P)
Purple Carrot Juice, p. 163	mineral water, non-carbonated, no flavour	green tea	coffee (P)
Cucumber and Mint Juice, p. 161	water, plain filtered or from a spring	milk, dairy, processed	cordial (P)
liquid chlorophyll; Green Water, p. 164	vegetable juice, packaged (MSG)	mineral water, carbonated, no flavour	dried soup mixes (MSG, P)
Anti-ageing Broth, p. 176		rice milk, plain (GI)	soft drink (sodas), flavoured (P)
		soy milk, plain organic	tap water
		tomato juice (MSG)	

Fruit

Strongly alkalising	Alkalising	Acidifying	Strongly acidifying
grapefruit	apricot, dried	apple, raw	blackcurrant
lemon	avocado	apricot, raw	blackthorn berry
lime	banana, dried (P)	blueberry	kiwi fruit
Flaxseed Lemon Drink, p. 165	banana, raw	cherries	mandarin
	date, dried (GI)	dried fruits, most (maybe MSG)	orange
	raisins (MSG)	fig, fresh & dried	mulberry
	tomato, raw (MSG)	grapes (MSG)	nectarine
		mango, fresh & dried	pineapple
		papaya	
		pawpaw	
		pear	
		persimmon	
		plum (MSG)	
		pomegranate	
		prunes (MSG)	
		raspberries	
		strawberries	
		tomato, cooked (MSG)	
		watermelon (GI)	

Vegetables

Strongly alkalising	Alkalising	Acidifying	Strong acidifying
barley grass (G)	artichoke	bamboo shoots	corn (grain)
beet greens, raw	asparagus	pea (legume) (MSG)	pickled gherkin
beetroot, beets, raw (GI)	brussels sprouts	pea, dried (legume)	pickled vegetables (in vinegar)
broccoli (MSG)	cabbage		
cucumber	carrot		
dandelion greens	capsicum (pepper)		
dark leafy greens, raw	cauliflower		
kale, raw	celery		
parsley	chicory		
rocket (arugula)	Chinese greens		
spinach, raw (MSG)	eggplant (aubergine)		
sprouts: alfalfa	garlic		
sprouts: lentil	green beans		
sprouts: mung bean	leek		
sprouts: snow pea (mangetout)	lettuce		
vegetable juice, fresh	marrow		
watercress	mushrooms (MSG)		
wheatgrass juice	olives		
	onion		
	pumpkin (winter squash)		
	silver beet, cooked (MSG)		
	snow peas (mangetout)		
	spring onion (shallot, scallion)		
	spinach, cooked (MSG)		
	swede (rutabaga)		
	turnip		
	zucchini (courgette)		

Note: potatoes are in the carbohydrate chart.

Carbohydrates: potatoes, grains, flours + breads

Strongly alkalising	Alkalising	Acidifying	Strongly acidifying
	potato, Carisma (low GI: available Australia, NZ)	barley (G)	corn
	potato, new	brown rice (GI)	corn cakes (corn crackers)
	potato, red (GI)	buckwheat	corn chips, tacos
	potato, white (GI)	oats, rolled (G)	corn flakes (GI)
	sweet potato	quinoa (GI: add cinnamon)	cornflour (GI)
	sprouted grains	rice milk, plain (GI)	millet (GI)
	sprouted bread (G)	pumpernickel (G)	pasta, white, wheat (G)
		rye flour (G)	polenta (GI)
		soy flour	processed wheat cereals (GI, G)
		spelt pasta (G)	white rice, jasmine (GI)
		spelt sourdough bread (G)	basmati rice, Doongara rice
		wholegrain bread (G)	white bread (GI, G)
		wholegrain wheat (G)	white flour, wheat (GI, G)
			yeast breads (G)

Nuts, seeds, oils + fats

Strongly alkalising	Alkalising	Acidifying	Strongly acidifying
	almonds	cashews, roasted	hazelnuts
	almond milk	coconut	hydrogenated fats
	Brazil nut (good source of selenium)	cold-pressed oils, heated	lard
	butter, pure (no additives to soften)	safflower oil	margarine (P)
	cold-pressed oils (unrefined, unheated), extra virgin olive oil and coconut oil	sesame seeds	peanuts
		sunflower oil	peanut oil
	linseeds Ω		pecans
	flaxseed oil Ω		pistachios
			pumpkin seeds
			sunflower seeds
			walnuts

Condiments, sweeteners, sweets, salt + spices

Strongly alkalising	Alkalising	Acidifying	Strongly acidifying
apple cider vinegar	calcium and magnesium	honey, processed	artificial sweetener (P)
	Celtic sea salt, unrefined sea salt (no anti-caking agent)	hydrolysed vegetable protein (MSG)	caramels, toffee
		tamari, wheat-free soy sauce (MSG)	chewing gum (P)
	cinnamon	soy sauce (MSG, G)	cocoa, chocolate (P)
	ginger	stock cubes (MSG)	glazed fruit (P)
	herbal medicines, various	vanilla essence	gravy (MSG)
	lecithin granules, soy	organic tomato sauce (MSG)	golden syrup
	Almond Pesto, p. 157		maple syrup, imitation
	rice malt syrup		mayonnaise (P)
	saffron		meat extracts (MSG)
	spices, all		mustard
	vanilla, whole bean		pickles
	potassium (mineral)		potato chips/crisps
	Beetroot and Almond Dip, p. 156		salt, table/processed
	Halo Dressing, p. 154		sugar, white
			sugar, raw/ brown
			tomato paste (MSG)
			tomato sauce, ketchup (MSG)
			vinegar, other

Protein: legumes, dairy, seafood, poultry + red meat

Strongly alkalising	Alkalising	Acidifying	Strongly acidifying
	egg yolk	anchovy	beef
		broad (fava) beans	bacon
		chicken (no skin)	butter, heated
		chick peas (garbanzo)	cheese
		egg whites	custard
		egg, whole, cooked	fish, dried, pickled, smoked, salted
		fish: trout, tuna, sardine Ω	herring Ω
		fish, fresh white (p. 68 for low mercury list) Ω	ice-cream (P)
		kidney beans	kefir (fermented milk)
		lamb	lobster
		lentils	meat pies (MSG)
		navy beans	mackerel Ω (mercury)
		oysters	peanuts
		peas (MSG)	pork, incl. ham
		soybeans, cooked	processed deli meats, seasoned, devon, salami etc. (MSG)
		soy milk, plain organic (G)	salmon Ω
		tuna, canned, in springwater	salmon, smoked Ω
		white (cannellini) beans	sausages (MSG)
		veal	yoghurt, sweetened

Resources

Karen Fischer's websites

www.healthbeforebeauty.com

www.theeczemadiet.com

www.eczemadiet.com.au

Further reading

Timeless Makeup: A step-by-step guide to looking younger, Rae Morris, Allen & Unwin

The Eczema Diet: Eczema-safe food to stop the itch and prevent eczema for life, Karen Fischer, Exisle Publishing

The Healthy Skin Diet: Your complete guide to beautiful skin in only 8 weeks, Karen Fischer, Exisle Publishing

The AGE-less Way: Escape America's overeating epidemic, Helen Vlassara

If you choose to change your supplement and skin care routine, the following is a sample of brands to help you get started. Please note I do not personally endorse or sell the following skin care and supplement brands and cannot vouch for quality and skin type suitability. Brand formulas can change after the printing of this book and there may be other brands that are more suited to your skin type and budget, and doing additional research of your own is recommended. See the review websites and if possible test products before buying.

Skin care product review websites
Make-up Alley
www.makeupalley.com

Supplements

Please check ingredients to ensure you don't double-up on nutrients. I have listed two examples of supplement combinations:

SUPPLEMENT ROUTINE 1

Take chromium, calcium citrate, vitamin D, magnesium and collagen-building nutrients zinc, manganese, silica, copper, vitamin C and iron.

Radiance 'Calcium Complex'
contains calcium, chromium, magnesium, vitamin D, zinc, iron, copper, silica, manganese (New Zealand)

OR Nature's Own 'Chromium Picolinate'
www.naturesown.com.au (available in Australia and New Zealand)

AND Cabot Health 'Calcium Complete'
contains calcium, magnesium, vitamin D, manganese, zinc and copper
www.cabothealth.com.au (Australia)

OR Blackmores 'Total Calcium + Magnesium + D3'
contains calcium, magnesium, vitamin D, manganese and zinc (no copper)
www.blackmores.com.au (Australia)
www.blackmoresnz.co.nz (New Zealand)

OR a powder formula if you can't swallow large tablets ...
BioMedica 'Bio Activated Calcium Powder'
prescription only; contains calcium, magnesium, vitamin D, zinc, manganese and vitamin C
www.biomedica.com.au (Australia)

AND Salus/Floradix 'Floravital Herbal Liquid Iron Extract'

gluten-free plant-based iron supplement if you have iron deficiency or anemia, or if you are a woman, vegetarian or vegan

www.salusuk.com (UK)

www.salus-haus.com/44/0/countries.html (other countries)

SUPPLEMENT ROUTINE 2

I am bringing out a beauty supplement range containing calcium, chromium, vitamin D, magnesium, collagen-building nutrients, and more, for younger skin. Refer to www.healthbeforebeauty.com for further details.

Skin care

Please check each website for shipping and availability in your country. Note that some products may also be stocked by your local beautician or available in your local health food shop or department store.

Avalon Organics

www.avalonorganics.com.au/storeloc.html (Australia)

www.avalonorganics.com (USA)

Colorescience

www.colorescience.com (USA)

Eco Logical Skin Care

www.ecologicalskin.com (Canada, USA and UK)

www.vitalenatural.com.au (Australia)

Environ

www.environskincareaustralia.com.au (Australia)

www.environ.co.za (South Africa and other countries)

John Plunkett

www.plunketts.com.au/superfade.html (Australia)

www.plunketts.com.au/stockists.html (stockists in Australia, New Zealand and Asia)

Jurlique

www.jurlique.com

La Mav Organic Skin Science (samples available)

www.lamav.com (Australia, New Zealand, Canada, USA, China, Japan etc.)

One Skin System (trial pack available)

www.oneskinsystem.com.au (Australia and New Zealand)

100 Percent Pure

www.100percentpure.com (USA)

REN Clean Skincare

www.renskincare.com (UK)

www.meccacosmetica.com.au/Ren (Australia)

Skinstitut

www.skinstitut.com (Australia, New Zealand)

Synergie and Synergie Minerals

www.synergieminerals.com (Australia, Canada, New Zealand, Hong Kong and Thailand)

Yes to Carrots; Yes to Blueberries

www.yestocarrots.com/find-a-store-australia.html (store locator Australia)

http://www.yestocarrots.com/find-a-store-uk.html (store locator UK)

www.yestocarrots.com (USA)

Acknowledgments

Writing books is such a privilege and I thank Gareth and Benny St John Thomas at Exisle Publishing for making that possible. So many people work together to make a book happen and my books are better thanks to editing by Anouska Jones and Karen Gee who have a passion for and an understanding of health. Thanks also to Tracey Gibbs for making this book look beautiful.

The ever-growing supply of science and nutritional biochemistry information has helped me to write this book and to look after my own skin. So I thank the researchers, scientists and doctors who make their research available to others, and a special thank you to Dr Jaime Uribarri, Professor of Medicine at the Mount Sinai School of Medicine in New York, for kindly answering my questions on AGEs. I'd also like to thank the skin care companies who help us to turn back time. It all helps!

Intuition is valuable too, and that brought me to Selwa Anthony, the writer's agent who I thank for helping to make my dream job become a reality. I'm lucky to have my children and they are often the first to test my recipes (in the early experimental stages — sorry and thank you!). And I'm grateful for the love and support from my mum and dad.

And to you — thank you for reading and for striving for better health. May you have younger and more beautiful skin very soon.

Warm wishes,

Karen

Endnotes

Introduction

1. Baldwin, J., 'The Fountain of Youth', 'Thirty more famous stories retold', retrieved 15 August 2012: http://www.mainlesson.com/display.php?-author=baldwin&book=thirty&story=fountain&PHPSESSID=860b-de18a074926abcb60146585b041b

2. 'Ponce de Leon discovers Florida', 'This day in history', retrieved 20 August 2012: http://www.history.com/this-day-in-history/ponce-de-leon-discovers-florida

3. Baldwin, J., loc. cit.

4. Tickner, F.J. and Medvei, V.C., 1958, 'Scurvy and the health of European crews in the Indian Ocean in the 17th century', *Medical History*, vol. 2, pp. 36–46.

5. Schlueter, A.K. and Johnston, C.S., 2011, 'Vitamin C: Overview and update', *Journal of Evidence-Based Complementary & Alternative Medicine*, vol. 16, no. 49, pp. 49–55.

6. Eileen Clark, Lawrence Scerri, 2008, 'Superficial and medium-depth chemical peels', *Clinics in Dermatology*, vol. 26, no. 2, pp. 209–18.

7. Popovich, D., et al., 2009, 'Scurvy forgotten but definitely not gone', *Journal of Pediatric Health Care*, vol. 23, no. 6, pp. 405–15.

Chapter 1

1. Boelsma, E. et al., 2003, 'Human skin condition and its associations with nutrient concentrations in serum and diet', *American Journal of Clinical Nutrition*, vol. 77, pp. 348–55.

2. ibid.

3. Baumann, L., 2007, 'Skin ageing and its treatment', *Journal of Pathology*, vol. 211, no. 2, pp. 241–51.

4. Verdier-Sévrain, S. et al., 2006, 'Biology of estrogens in skin: Implications for skin aging', *Experimental Dermatology*, vol. 15, pp. 83–94.

5. Sumino, H. et al., 2004, 'Effects of aging, menopause and hormone replacement on forearm skin elasticity in women', *Journal of the American Geriatrics Society*, vol. 52, no. 6, pp. 945–9.

Chapter 2

1. Baumann, L., 2007, 'Skin ageing and its treatment', *Journal of Pathology*, vol. 211, no. 2, pp. 241–51.

2. Danby, F.W., 2010, 'Nutrition and aging skin: Sugar and glycation', *Clinics in Dermatology*, vol. 28, no. 4, pp. 409–11.

3. Luevano-Contreras, C. et al., 2010, 'Dietary advanced glycation end products and aging', *Nutrients*, vol. 2, pp. 1247–65.

4. Kuwabara, T., 2010, 'The changes in optical properties of skin related to carbonylation of proteins in the horny layer', Proceedings of the 11th Annual Meeting of Japanese Photo-Aging Research Society, p. 29.

5. Ohshima, H. et al., 2009, 'Melanin and facial skin fluorescence as markers of yellowish discoloration with aging', *Skin Research and Technology*, vol. 15, pp. 496–502.

6. Ichihashi, M. et al., 2011, 'Glycation stress and photo-aging in skin', *Anti-Aging Medicine*, vol. 8, no. 3, pp. 23–9.

7. Tang, S.Y. et al., 2007, 'Effects of non-enzymatic glycation on cancellous bone fragility', *Bone*, vol. 40, pp. 1144–51.

8. Luevano-Contreras, C. et al., 2010, loc. cit.

9. Danby, F.W., 2010, loc. cit.

10. Kuwabara, T., 2010, loc. cit.

11. Ohshima, H. et al., 2009, loc. cit.

12. Ichihashi, M. et al., 2011, loc. cit.

13. Luevano-Contreras, C. et al., 2010, loc. cit.

14. ibid.

15. ibid.

16. Palmer, D.M. and Silverman Kitchin, J., 2010, 'Oxidative damage, skin aging, antioxidants and a novel antioxidant rating system', *Journal of Drugs in Dermatology*, vol. 9, no. 1, pp. 11–5.

17. ibid.

18. Pepper, E.D. et al., 2010, 'Antiglycation effects of carnosine and other compounds on the long-term survival of escherichia coli', *Applied and Environmental Microbiology*, vol. 76, no. 24, pp. 7925–30.

19. Babizhayev, M.A. et al., 2012, 'Skin beautification with oral non-hydrolized versions of carnosine and carcinine: Effective therapeutic management and cosmetic skincare solutions against oxidative glycation and free-radical production as a causal mechanism of diabetic complications and skin aging', *Journal of Dermatological Treatment*, vol. 23, no. 5, pp. 345–84.

20. Thirunavukkarasu, V. et al., 2005, 'Lipoic acid prevents collagen abnormalities in tail tendon of high-fructose-fed rats', *Diabetes, Obesity and Metabolism*, vol. 7, no. 3, pp. 294–7.

21. Dearlove, R.P. et al., 2008, 'Inhibition of protein glycation by extracts of culinary herbs and spices', *Journal of Medicinal Food*, vol. 11, no. 2, pp. 275–81.

22. Wu, C.H. and Yen, G.C., 2005, 'Inhibitory effect of naturally occurring flavonoids on the formation of advanced glycation end products', *Journal of Agricultural and Food Chemistry*, vol. 53, pp. 3167–73.

Chapter 3

1. Luevano-Contreras, C. et al., 2010, loc. cit.

2. Lustig, R.H. et al., 2012, 'Public health: The toxic truth about sugar', *Nature*, vol. 482, no. 7383.

3. Danby, F.W., 2010, loc. cit.

4. ibid.

5. Monnier, V.M. et al., 2006, 'Cross-linking of the extracellular matrix by the Maillard Reaction in aging and diabetes: An update on "a puzzle nearing resolution"', *Annals of the New York Academy of Sciences*, vol. 1043, no. 1, pp. 533–44.

6. Stanton, R., 2007, *Rosemary Stanton's Complete Book of Food and Nutrition*, Simon & Schuster.

7. Hall, W.L. et al., 2003, 'Physiological mechanisms mediating aspartame-induced satiety', *Physiol Behav*, vol. 78, no. 4–5, pp. 557–62.

8. Sies, H. and Stahl, W., 2004, 'Nutritional protection against skin damage from sunlight', *Annual Review of Nutrition*, vol. 24, pp. 173–200.

9. Danby, F.W., 2010, loc. cit.

10. Bernstein, E.F., Underhill, C.B., Hahn, P.J., Brown, D.B. and Uitto, J., 1996, 'Chronic sun exposure alters both the content and distribution of dermal glycosaminoglycans', *British Journal of Dermatology*, vol. 135, no. 2, pp. 255–62.

11. Sies, H., 2004, loc. cit.

12. ibid.

13. Purba, M., et al. 2001, 'Skin wrinkling: can food make a difference?' *Journal of the American College of Nutrition*, vol. 20, no. 1, pp 71–80.

14. Uribarri, J. et al., 2010, 'Advanced gycation end products in foods and a practical guide to their reduction in the diet', *Journal of the American Dietetic Association*, vol. 110, no. 6, pp. 911–6.

15. ibid.

16. ibid.

17. Bingham, S.A, Pignatelli, B., Pollock, J.R. et al., 1996, 'Does increased endogenous formation of N-nitroso compounds in the human colon explain the association between red meat and colon cancer?', *Carcinogenesis*, vol. 17, no. 3, pp. 515–23.

18. Chong, E.W.T. et al., 2008, 'Red meat and chicken consumption and its association with age-related macular degeneration', *American Journal of Epidemiology*, vol. 169, no. 7, pp. 867.

19. ibid.

20. Pan, A. et al., 2012, 'Red meat consumption and mortality: Results from 2 prospective cohort studies', *Archives of Internal Medicine*, vol. 172, no. 7, pp. 555–63.

21. ibid.

22. ibid.

23. Table adapted from Uribarri, J. et al., 2010, 'Advanced gycation end products in foods and a practical guide to their reduction in the diet', *Journal of the American Dietetic Association*, vol. 110, no. 6, pp. 911–6.

24. Uribarri, J. et al., 2010, loc. cit.

25. Purba, M., 2001, loc. cit.

26. Adebamowo, C.A. et al., 2005, 'High school dietary dairy intake and teenage acne', *Journal of the American Academy of Dermatology*, vol. 52, no. 2, pp 360–2.

27. Uribarri, J. et al., 2010, loc. cit.

28. Vander Straten, M. et al., 2001, 'Tobacco use and skin disease', *Southern Medical Journal*, vol. 94, no. 6, pp. 621–34.

29. Saavedra, J.M., Harris, G.D. and Finberg, L., 1991, 'Capillary refilling (skin turgor) in the assessment of dehydration', *American Journal of Diseases of Children*, vol. 145, no. 3, pp. 296–98.

30. Vander Straten, M. et al., 2001, loc. cit.

31. Sarin, C.L., Austin, J.C. and Nickel, W.O., 1974, *Journal of the American Medical Association*, vol. 229, in Vander Straten M. et al, 2001, 'Tobacco use and skin disease', *Southern Medical Journal*.

32. Luevano-Contreras, C. et al., 2010, loc. cit.

33. Vander Straten, M. et al., 2001, loc. cit.

34. Sarin, C.L., Austin, J.C. and Nickel, W.O., 1974, loc. cit.

35. Freiman, A. et al., 2004, 'Cutaneous effects of smoking', *Journal of Cutaneous Medicine and Surgery*, vol. 8, no. 6, pp. 415–23.

36. ibid.

37. Emery, C.F. et al., 2005, 'Exercise accelerates wound healing among healthy older adults: A preliminary investigation', *Journal of Gerontology*, vol. 60A, no. 11, pp. 1432–6.

38. Boor, P. et al., 2009, Regular moderate exercise reduces advanced glycation and ameliorates early diabetic nephropathy in obese Zucker rats', *Metabolism Clinical and Experimental*, vol. 58, pp. 1669–77.

39. Emery, C.F. et al., 2005, loc. cit.

40. Boor, P. et al., 2009, loc. cit.

41. Marta, K. et al., 2004, 'Advanced glycation end-products in patients with chronic alcohol misuse', *Alcohol and Alcoholism*, vol. 39, no. 4, pp. 316–20.

42. ibid.

43. ibid.

44. ibid.

45. Lewis, S. et al., 2008, 'Alcohol as a cause of cancer', Cancer Institute NSW Monograph, retrieved 12 August 2009: http://www.cancerinstitute.org.au/cancer_inst/publications/pdfs/pm–2008–03_alcohol–as–a–cause–of–cancer.pdf

46. Uribarri, J. et al., 2010, loc. cit.

47. ibid.

48. ibid.

49. Liu, S. et al., 2003, 'Is intake of breakfast cereals related to total and cause-specific mortality in men?', *American Journal of Clinical Nutrition*, vol. 77, no. 3, pp. 594–9.

50. Pan, A. et al., 2012, loc. cit.

51. Chong, E.W.T. et al., 2008, loc. cit.

52. Sausenthaler, S. et al., 2006, 'Margarine and butter consumption, eczema and allergic sensitization in children', *Pediatric Allergy and Immunology*, vol. 17, no. 2, pp. 85–93.

53. Bolte, G, et al., 2001, 'Margarine consumption and allergy in children', *American Journal of Respiratory and Critical Care Medicine*, vol. 163, pp. 277–9.

54. Uribarri, J. et al., 2010, loc. cit.

55. Uribarri, J. et al., 2010, loc. cit.

56. Gugliucci, A. et al., 2009, 'Short-term low calorie diet intervention reduces serum advanced glycation end products in healthy overweight or obese adults', *Annals of Nutrition and Metabolism*, vol. 54, no. 3, pp. 197–201.

57. Uribarri, J. and Tuttle, K.R., 2006, 'Advanced glycation end products and nephrotoxicity of high-protein diets', *Clinical Journal of the American Society of Nephrology*, vol. 1, no. 6, pp. 1293–9.

58. Gugliucci, A. et al., 2009, loc cit.

59. Vlassara, H. et al. 2009, 'Protection against loss of innate defenses in adulthood by low advanced glycation end products (AGE) intake: Role of the anti-inflammatory AGE receptor-1', *Journal of Clinical Endocrinology & Metabolism,* vol. 94, no. 11, pp. 4483–91.

60. Uribarri, J. et al., 2010, loc. cit.

Chapter 4

1. Boniface, R. and Robert, A.M., 1996, 'Effect of anthocyanins on human connective tissue metabolism in the human', *Klin Monbl Augenheilkd*, vol. 209, no. 6, pp. 368–72.

2. Kowalczyk, E. et al., 2003, 'Anthocyanins in medicine', *Polish Journal of Pharmacology*, vol. 55, pp. 699–702.

3. Vinson, J.A. and Howard, H.B., 1996, 'Inhibition of protein glycation and advanced glycation end products by ascorbic acid and other vitamins and nutrients', *Journal of Nutritional Biochemistry*, vol. 7, pp. 659–63.

4. Draelos, Z.D., Yatskayer, M., Raab, S. and Oresajo, C., 2009, 'An evaluation of the effect of a topical product containing C-xyloside and blueberry extract on the appearance of type II diabetic skin', *J Cosmet Dermatol*, vol. 8, pp. 147–51.

5. Mizutani, K. et al., 2000, 'Resveratrol inhibits AGEs-induced proliferation and collagen synthesis activity in vascular smooth muscle cells from stroke-prone spontaneously hypertensive rats', *Biochemical and Biophysical Research Communications*, vol. 274, no. 1, pp. 61–7.

6. Wang, W. et al., 2011, 'Phytochemicals from berries and grapes inhibited the formation of advanced glycation end-products by scavenging reactive carbonyls', *Food Research International*, vol. 44, no., 9, pp. 2666–73.

7. Draelos, Z.D., Yatskayer, M., Raab, S. and Oresajo, C., 2009, loc. cit.

8. Gupta, S. and Mukhtar, H., 2002, 'Chemoprevention of skin cancer: Current status and future prospects', *Cancer and Metastasis Reviews*, vol. 21, no. 3, pp. 363–80.

9. Perez-Vicente, A. et al., 2002, 'In vitro gastrointestinal digestion study of pomegranate juice phenolic compounds, anthocyanins and vitamin C', *Journal of Agricultural and Food Chemistry*, vol. 50, pp. 2308–12.

10. Gil, M.I. et al., 2000, 'Antioxidant activity of pomegranate juice and its relationship with phenolic composition and processing', *Journal Agricultural and Food Chemistry*, vol. 48, pp. 4581–9.

11. Puppala, M. and Chandrasekhar, A., 2012, 'Ellagic acid, a new antiglycating agent: its inhibition of N lunate epsilon-(carboxymethyl) lysine', *Biochemical Journal*, vol. 442, no. 1, pp. 221–30.

12. Muthenna, P. et al., 2012, 'Ellagic acid, a new antiglycating agent: Its inhibition of Nε-(carboxymethyl)lysine', *Biochemical Journal*, vol. 442, pp. 221–30.

13. Umadevi, S. et al., 2012, 'Studies on the cardio protective role of gallic acid against AGE-induced cell proliferation and oxidative stress in H9C2 (2-1) cells', *Cardiovascular Toxicology*, vol. 12, no. 4, pp. 304–11.

14. Fossen, T. et al., 1998, 'Flavonoids from red onion (Allium cepa)', *Phytochemistry*, vol. 47, no. 2, pp. 281–5.

15. Shon, Mi-Yae et al., 2004, 'Antimutagenic, antioxidant and free radical scavenging activity of ethyl acetate extracts from white, yellow and red onions', *Food and Chemical Toxicology*, vol. 42, no. 4, pp. 659–66.

16. Peijun, M. et al., 1998, 'Blocking effect of quercetin on the nonenzymatic glycation of aortic collagen', *Chinese Journal of Diabetes*, vol. 1, pp. 10.

17. Kim, H.Y. and Kim, K., 2003, 'Protein glycation inhibitory and antioxidative activities of some plant extracts in vitro', *Journal of Agricultural and Food Chemistry*, vol. 51, no. 6, pp. 1586–91.

18. Thaipong, K. et al., 2006, 'Comparison of ABTS, DPPH, FRAP, and ORAC assays for estimating antioxidant activity from guava fruit extracts', *Journal of Food Composition and Analysis*, vol. 19, pp. 669–75.

19. Huang, C.S. et al., 2011, 'Antihyperglycemic and antioxidative potential of Psidium guajava fruit in streptozotocin-induced diabetic rats', *Food and Chemical Toxicology*, vol. 49, pp. 2189–95.

20. Wu, J.W. et al., 2009, 'Inhibitory effects of guava (Psidium guajava L.) leaf extracts and its active compounds on the glycation process of protein', *Food Chemistry*, vol. 113, no. 1, pp. 78–84.

21. Huang, C.S. et al., 2011, loc. cit.

22. Nishad Fathima, N. et al., 2009, 'Collagen–curcumin interaction — A physico-chemical study', *Journal of Chemical Sciences*, vol. 121, no. 4, pp. 509–14.

23. Sajithlal, G.B. et al., 1998, 'Effect of curcumin on the advanced glycation and cross-linking of collagen in diabetic rats', *Biochemical Pharmacology*, vol. 56, no. 12, pp. 1607–14.

24. Nishad Fathima, N. et al., 2009, loc. cit.

25. Jagtap, A.G. and Patil, P.B., 2010, 'Antihyperglycemic activity and inhibition of advanced glycation end product formation by Cuminum cyminum in streptozotocin induced diabetic rats', *Food and Chemical Toxicology*, vol. 48, no. 8, pp. 2030–36.

26. Shanmugam, K. R. et al., 2011, 'Neuroprotective effect of ginger on anti-oxidant enzymes in streptozotocin-induced diabetic rats', *Food and Chemical Toxicology*, vol. 49, no. 4, pp. 893–7.

27. Dearlove, R.P. et al., 2008, loc. cit.

28. Milind, P. and Deepa, K., 2011, 'Clove: A champion spice', *Journal of Research in Ayurveda and Pharmacy*, vol. 2, no. 1, pp. 47–54.

29. Lee, Y.Y. et al., 2007, 'Eugenol suppressed the expression of lipopolysaccharide-induced proinflammatory mediators in human macrophages', *Journal of Endodontics*, vol. 33, no. 6, pp. 698–702.

30. Ranasinghe, P. et al., 2012, 'Effects of *Cinnamomum zeylanicum* (Ceylon cinnamon) on blood glucose and lipids in diabetic and healthy rat model', *Pharmacognosy Research*, vol. 4, no. 2, pp. 73–9.

31. Ramful, D. et al., 2010, 'Citrus fruit extracts reduce advanced glycation end products (AGEs)- and H2O2-induced oxidative stress in human adipocytes', *Journal of Agricultural and Food Chemistry*, vol. 58, pp. 11119–29.

32. Uribarri, J. et al., 2010, loc. Cit.

33. Ray, R.C. et al., 2011, 'Anti-oxidant properties and other functional attributes of tomato: An overview', *International Journal of Food and Fermentation Technology*, vol. 1, no. 2, pp. 139–48.

34. ibid.

Chapter 5

1. Johnston, C.S. and Gaas, C.A., 2006, 'Vinegar: Medicinal uses and antiglycemic effect', *Medscape General Medicine*, vol. 8, no. 2, p. 61.

2. Hlebowicz, J. et al., 2007, 'Effect of apple cider vinegar on delayed gastric emptying in patients with type 1 diabetes mellitus: A pilot study', *BMC Gastroenterology*, vol. 7, p. 46.

3. Ireland, C, 'Hormones in milk can be dangerous', *Harvard University Gazette*, 7 Dec 2006.

4. De Spirt, S. et al., 2009, 'Intervention with flaxseed and borage oil supplements modulates skin condition in women', *British Journal of Nutrition*, vol. 101, no. 3, p. 440.

5. Farahpour, M.R. et al., 2011, 'Wound healing activity of flaxseed Linum usitatissimum L. in rats', *African Journal of Pharmacy and Pharmacology*, vol. 5, no. 21, pp. 2386–9.

6. Neukam, K. et al., 2011, 'Supplementation of flaxseed oil diminishes skin sensitivity and improves skin barrier function and condition', *Skin Pharmacology and Physiology*, vol. 24, no. 2, 67–74.

Chapter 6

1. Denda, M., Hosoi, J., and Asida, Y., 2000, 'Visual imaging of ion distribution in human epidermis', *Biochemical and Biophysical Research Communications*, vol. 272, no. 1, pp. 134-7.

2. Denda, M., 2000, 'Skin barrier function as a self-organizing system', *Forma*, vol. 15, no. 3, pp. 227-32.

3. Purba, M., et al. 2001, 'Skin wrinkling: can food make a difference?' *Journal of the American College of Nutrition*, vol. 20, no. 1, pp. 71–80.

4. Vinson, J.A. and Howard, H.B., 1996, loc. cit.

5. Boelsma, E. et al., 2003, loc. cit.

6. Hodges, R.E. et al. 1969, 'Experimental scurvy in man', *American Journal of Clinical Nutrition*, vol. 22, no. 5, pp 535–48.

7. ibid.

8. Jugdaohsingh, R. et al., 2002, 'Dietary silicon intake and absorption', *American Journal of Clinical Nutrition*, vol. 75, no. 5, pp. 887–93.

Chapter 7

1. Kafi, R. et al., 2007, 'Improvement of naturally aged skin with vitamin A (retinol)', *Archives of Dermatology*, vol. 143, no. 5, pp. 606–12.

2. ibid.

3. Garg, V.K. et al., 2008, 'Glycolic acid peels versus salicylic-mandelic acid peels in active acne vulgaris and post-acne scarring and hyperpigmentation: A comparative study', *Dermatologic Surgery*, vol. 35, no. 1, pp. 59–65.

4. Fartasch, M., et al., 1997, 'Mode of action of glycolic acid on human stratum corneum: Ultrastructural and functional evaluation of the epidermal barrier', *Archives of Dermatological Research*, vol. 289, no. 7, pp. 404–409.

5. Fuchs, K.O. et al., 2003, 'The effects of an estrogen and glycolic acid cream on the facial skin of postmenopausal women: A randomized histologic study', *Change*, vol. 70, pp. 3–7.

6. Kim, S.J. and Won, Y.H., 1998, 'The effect of glycolic acid on cultured human skin fibroblasts: Cell proliferative effect and increased collagen synthesis', *Journal of Dermatology*, vol. 25, no. 2, p. 85.

7. Mizutani, K. et al., 2000, 'Resveratrol inhibits AGEs-induced proliferation and collagen synthesis activity in vascular smooth muscle cells from stroke-prone spontaneously hypertensive rats', *Biochemical and Biophysical Research Communications*, vol. 274, no. 1, pp. 61–7.

8. Gupta, S. and Mukhtar, H. 2002, 'Chemoprevention of skin cancer: Current status and future prospects', *Cancer and Metastasis Reviews*, vol. 21, no. 3, pp. 363–80.

9. Baxter, R.A., 2008, 'Anti-aging properties of resveratrol: Review and

report of a potent new antioxidant skin care formulation', *Journal of Cosmetic Dermatology*, vol. 7, no. 1, pp. 2–7.

10. ibid.

11. Mizutani, K. et al., 2000, loc. cit.

12. Gupta, S. and Mukhtar, H. 2002, loc. cit.

13. Humbert, P.G. et al., 2003, 'Topical ascorbic acid on photoaged skin. Clinical, topographical and ultrastructural evaluation: Double-blind study vs. placebo', *Experimental Dermatology*, vol. 12, no. 3, pp. 237–44.

14. Fitzpatrick R.E. and Rostan E.F., 2002, 'Double-blind, half-face study comparing topical vitamin C and vehicle for rejuvenation of photodamage', *Dermatologic Surgery*, vol. 28, no. 3, pp. 231–6.

15. Colven, R.M. and Pinnell, S.R., 1996, 'Topical vitamin C in aging', *Clinics in Dermatology*, vol. 14, no. 2, p. 227.

16. ibid.

17. Etcoff, N.L. et al., 2011, 'Cosmetics as a feature of the extended human phenotype: Modulation of the perception of biologically important facial signals', *PloS One*, vol. 6, no. 10, e25656.

18. ibid.

Chapter 8

1. Boor, P. et al., 2009, loc. cit.

2. Emery, C.F. et al., 2005, loc. cit.

3. Danby, F.W., 2010, loc. cit.

4. Sarıfakıoglu, N. et al., 2004, 'A new phenomenon: "Sleep lines" on the face"', *Scandinavian Journal of Plastic and Reconstructive Surgery and Hand Surgery*, vol. 38, no. 4, pp. 244–7.

5. Kripke, D.F. et al., 2002, 'Mortality associated with sleep duration and insomnia', *Archives of General Psychiatry*, vol. 59, no. 2, p. 131.

6. Butler, S.T., 2011, 'Sun hazards in your car', *Skin Cancer Foundation Journal*, vol. XXIX, pp. 94–6.

7. ibid.

8. Voelkle, M.C. et al., 2012, 'Let me guess how old you are: Effects of age, gender, and facial expression on perceptions of age', *Psychology and Aging*, vol. 27, no. 2, p. 265.

9. Nash, R. et al., 2006, 'Cosmetics: They influence more than Caucasian female facial attractiveness', *Journal of Applied Social Psychology*, vol. 36, no. 2, pp. 493–504.

AGE food list

1. Adapted from Table 1 in Uribarri, J. et al., 2010, 'Advanced gycation end products in foods and a practical guide to their reduction in the diet', *Journal of the American Dietetic Association*, vol. 110, no. 6, pp. 911–6.

Index

Also by Karen Fischer and Exisle Publishing ...

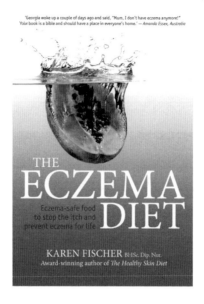

'Georgia woke up a couple of days ago and said, "Mum, I don't have eczema anymore!" Your book is a bible and should have a place in everyone's home.' — *Amanda Essex, Australia*

THE
ECZEMA
DIET
Eczema-safe food to stop the itch and prevent eczema for life

KAREN FISCHER BHSc. Dip. Nut.
Award-winning author of *The Healthy Skin Diet*

The Eczema Diet
Eczema-safe food to stop the itch and prevent eczema for life

For the first time, the findings of hundreds of international researchers and skin specialists have been pieced together to solve the eczema puzzle. The result is the first diet designed to correct the underlying causes of eczema so you can gradually go back to a normal diet and remain eczema-free.

Whether you have a mild patch of dermatitis or you're enduring chronic eczema from head to toe, *The Eczema Diet* shows you how to create beautiful skin for life. Tried and tested for more than a decade, the comprehensive program covers all eczema conditions and features separate programs catering for all age groups, including babies.

ISBN 978-1-921966-06-4

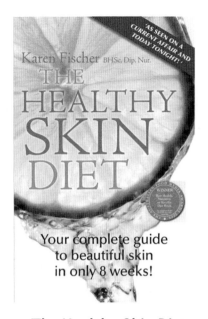

The Healthy Skin Diet
Your complete guide to beautiful skin in only 8 weeks!

Winner of the 2008 Australian Food Media Award for Best Health, Nutrition or Specific Diet Book, *The Healthy Skin Diet* offers an easy-to-follow, comprehensive program featuring planned daily menus; a three-day detox plan; delicious, simple, healthy, alkalising recipes; and chapters dedicated to the treatment of specific skin disorders. Whether you want to eliminate acne, cellulite, dandruff, dermatitis, eczema, psoriasis or rosacea, or simply fight the signs of ageing, the answers are in this book! Beautiful skin is not something exclusively reserved for the genetically blessed. You too can have great healthy, clear and blemish-free skin.

ISBN 978-1-921966-13-2

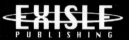